# The Good, the Bad, and the **Heavy**

## The BOLD Truth About Bodybuilding

### CHRIS HARRISON

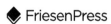

FriesenPress

Suite 300 - 990 Fort St
Victoria, BC, V8V 3K2
Canada

www.friesenpress.com

ISBN
978-1-5255-8904-1 (Hardcover)
978-1-5255-8905-8 (Paperback)
978-1-5255-8906-5 (eBook)

*1. HEALTH & FITNESS, EXERCISE*

Distributed to the trade by The Ingram Book Company

# Table of Contents

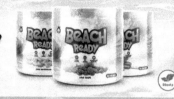
  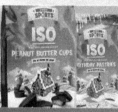
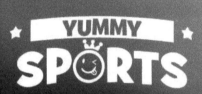
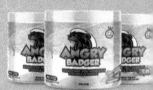
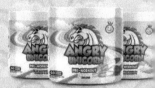
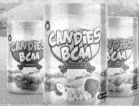
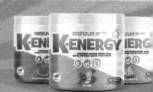

# Acknowledgements

First and foremost, I would like to thank you for taking the time to read though this book. I hope it will be informative and give you a well-rounded look into the sport of bodybuilding. Entering the sport competitively can be quite an intimidating and daunting challenge. I hope this gives you the knowledge to help you through your first contest preps. Once you compete a couple times you will start to get the hang of things.

If you are a friend or family member of an athlete competing in this sport, I thank you from the bottom of my heart for reading this. I wish a book like this had been available when I started with bodybuilding instead of learning things the hard way and having to show my loved ones what this sport really is about. Knowledge is power. The more we know before we begin this sport, the safer we will be. Protecting our health and safety is of the utmost importance so we can all enjoy a prolonged, safe, and robust career.

All I want is for people to enjoy the sport as much I do. This sport literally saved my life and I wouldn't be here without it. Even if I can motivate one person toward this sport and save them, my job is done.

Thank you, future athletes; thank you, family and friends; and thank you to anyone who reads this book. It means so much to me that you have made an effort to help yourself or one of your loved ones. We need more people like you in this sport and the world in general.

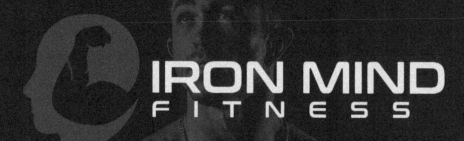

# IRON MIND
## F I T N E S S

# *BODY TRANSFORMATION SPECIALIST*

A healthier, fitter you is just around the corner

**Contact us on Instagram @Ironmfitness**

Personalized and affordable transformation packages. All include nutrition and training plans, weekly checkins, accountability, necessary adjustments and instant support

# Introduction

This book was developed as a teaching tool for not only new fitness athletes curious about the sport of bodybuilding, but also as an education tool for the friends and family closest to them that don't actually know the bold truth about bodybuilding.

Rather than going into a lot of detail about how the industry works, I'm going to keep things simple and precise. I want to paint a clear picture of what the life of a bodybuilder and fitness competitor actually is like. Some chapters and statements are going to apply to some people more than others, but the general idea remains the same. Everyone new to and entering the sport needs to know what they are about to get themselves into, from the good, the bad, the ugly, and everything in between.

In my experience, people in the fitness industry often have very little support from friends and family. There are many reasons for this.

Athletes continue to be beaten down by negative comments and the false accusations that people hear from mainstream media, and it gets to the point where athletes don't even want to try to talk about it anymore. Most, including myself, are sick of repeating themselves like a broken record, but here is the truth: Most of the "facts" that people have been hearing are, in fact, not true at all. Unfortunately, those words usually fall on deaf ears.

I truly believe that helping people understand the truth about the fitness and bodybuilding industry will not only help it grow exponentially, but also start to help eliminate the inaccuracies and misinformation that we have been struggling with since its inception. This book will not only give the athletes the support and knowledge they need to thrive, but it will also give friends and family the information necessary to help support and prepare them for the challenges both parties will likely inevitably encounter.

# Guests

You will be hearing from a few different people involved in various aspects of the industry. A top Canadian fitness and competition prep coach, an International Federation of Bodybuilding & Fitness (IFBB) pro, his wife and my own mother. This should give a well-balanced view of the fitness and bodybuilding world as we know it today.

I will admit, some of it will sound shocking and scary, but some will be much more pleasant. I'm not here to hide anything. I'm here to bring everyone the best, most diverse view of the sport of bodybuilding so that potential new athletes, friends, and family can fully understand what they're getting into and acknowledge what it's going to take from all parties to succeed in this spectacular sport.

I am convinced that opening up this kind of dialogue is what it's going to take to start growing this industry into a respectable and dominant sport that I believe it should be. A major problem lies with people living in fear about talking about the positive and negative aspects of this sport. Let's crack this egg open and let the truth spill out so we can all fully comprehend and enjoy this magnificent and beautiful sport.

## Ryan Richardson

Ryan Richardson is the owner and head coach of Team Ignite Fitness (Instagram: @teamignitefitness), one of Canada's leading fitness and contest prep teams in the country. He is an extremely successful, in-demand coach based out of Calgary, Alberta, with a ninety percent top five placing rate of his athletes. His athletes range from first-time competitors to IFBB pros. His experience and knowledge in the industry is extraordinary, which is why he is such a dominant figure in the fitness industry and why I chose him to be part of this literature.

## Karen Harrison

Who better to hear from then the woman who raised me? My mother, Karen Harrison, has been an ER nurse for over twenty years and has personally witnessed the nasty side that this sport has the potential to exhibit.

Learning from her son, she has also been able to see the beauty that tends to be overlooked in this sport, and is now able to approach the topic of bodybuilding from all angles. She has seen it all, the good, the bad, and the heavy.

With her medical and emergency background, plus having witnessed firsthand her son's struggles and triumphs in the industry, she is an amazing source of credible and superior information that I know you will take to heart.

## Alfred and Shauna Voit

If you want genuine and inside knowledge about living a life together inside the fitness industry, then Alfred and Shauna Voit are the people you need to listen to (Instagram: @alfredvphysique_ifbb_pro and @shaunavoit).

Alfred competed in thirteen shows in just under three years, eventually earning his professional status in 2018. As you can imagine, this kind of lifestyle can have its challenges when you are in a committed relationship. Especially when your partner isn't fully involved in the industry.

That being said, Shauna has recently competed in her very first competition and has had the opportunity to experience the lifestyle and the process from inside the looking glass. This not only makes her a fantastic source of information on how strenuous life can be living with a partner that's now a professional athlete, but also living a life on the other extreme as the athlete preparing to compete. I would highly recommend taking both of their experiences, perspectives, and knowledge to heart, as you will not be able to find information more valuable than this.

# Chapter 1:
# What is Bodybuilding?

Bodybuilding is probably the most difficult sport on this planet. There is no break in this industry. There is only focus, dedication, and hard work, and it takes its toll on the mind, body, and soul. Day in and day out, you will experience the difficulty of this industry and it only gets increasingly difficult the deeper you delve into it.

Just like tattoos, piercings, Botox, branding, breast implants, scarification, etc., bodybuilding at its core is a form of body modification. You are literally altering the body through a particular set of actions in order to change your physical appearance. It's all to change how you look, how people perceive you, and how you perceive yourself. It's that simple. If you're looking to gain muscle, lose a few pounds, or to tighten up for your vacation, you're participating in bodybuilding to an extent.

Bodybuilding as a profession, however, goes considerably deeper than that, almost to an unimaginable level. It can sometimes take up to twenty years to achieve dramatic results, and some people will never be satisfied with how they look. Bodybuilding is a marathon sport, it's not a sprint. Therefore, patience is of the utmost importance if one is to be a long-term player.

When it comes to fitness, you must decide what you want. That way you can make a plan for how to achieve those specific results, because a plan is essential to your success.

For example, a person that's looking to lose twenty, fifty, or one hundred pounds is going to take a completely different approach to get those results as a person looking to gain twenty, fifty, or one hundred pounds of muscle. Of course, there are different extents that someone can go to too get the results they are looking for. Some want to be massive muscle machines, others want to look more aesthetically pleasing and well balanced, and some people just want to look like they're in somewhat good shape.

Bodybuilding is a beautiful work of art in one of its purest forms. Just like a stunning painting or hand-crafted piece of carpentry, it takes a significant amount of skill, knowledge, time, and sacrifice to bring out the beauty in bodybuilding. While some people are using paint brushes and skill saws, bodybuilders are using tools such as weights, food, and supplements. The goal of looking and feeling like you've been carved from marble like a Greek god is real. That feeling you get when you're finally happy with how you look in the mirror is nothing other than pure ecstasy.

Unfortunately, like all other art forms, not all people can agree on what is beautiful and what is not. People must be aware of this. When you're a competitor, criticism in this industry can be absolutely insane, and it will crush you if you aren't prepared for it. People and judges won't be afraid to tell you their opinions of how you look in this sport.

From my experience in this sport, someone is always too fat, skinny, muscular, lean, tall, short, or whatever. All you can do is just take it with a grain of salt and ignore it. People are entitled to have their opinion, just like you are, but don't let it discourage you. You have goals to achieve, and the opinion of others is not worth giving up over. In fact, I've learned that when people start to try to pull you down, you are on the right path. Those who want to hold you back instead of pushing you forward are those who have negatively influenced you to become who you ultimately don't want to be to begin with. They have shown their true colours, and the decision to drop that relationship for your own happiness is likely in your best interest. I have had to do this on many occasions, even with family. Those who don't help push you toward your goals aren't worth your time.

When or if you or a loved one competes in the sport, keep in mind that this is whole new level of judgment. You are literally training to go onstage to be judged by a panel of other human beings. It can be mentally exhausting to handle. However, constructive criticism is a different story. Positive criticism is necessary to achieve the looks one needs for competition.

Take a second right now and imagine going onstage in your underwear in front of hundreds or thousands of strangers to pose your body to be judged, not only by the judging panel, but by the entire audience. It can be tough to deal with, and that's an understatement. You need to be mentally resilient to compete in bodybuilding, so be ready.

This is the only sport that truly requires you to be on a strict diet all year round, while consistently pushing your mental and physical capacities to their limits. Then, when you're in a pre-contest prep, you have to do all of this while cutting weight and living on a calorie deficit for months on end.

There isn't another sport on this planet that I can think of that requires this kind of work ethic while depleting the body to its extremes. It feels torturous, painful, and stressful. It's expensive, and it feels like it never ends. Your mental capability is going to be taken to its absolute limit every day, and it's going to freaking suck.

But when you see yourself or another committed athlete hit the stage in none other than extraordinary shape, you witness the sport's purity, grace, beauty, and elegance. The way different body types present themselves, the way you can see how the muscles contract and relax, you witness the body's ability to shine and take on a whole new appearance.

The artistry behind how people present their muscle groups to the audience can be breathtaking. Its magnificence all comes out in the five minutes you or someone else has onstage, and those are the very moments that you train for. The moment you unveil yourself to the world is the absolute best feeling you will ever experience in your life. It makes all the pain, plain food, early morning cardio, and painful weight training worth it.

# Bodybuilding Classes

Competitive bodybuilding has many different classes for all sorts of body types for both male and female competitors. Both male and female classes listed here can be further broken down into age groups if a competitor would like to compete with anyone of a similar age. These classes may vary, depending on where and in what federation a competitor decides to compete. Generally, these age groups are as follows:

- Open (Any age can compete together)
- Novice (23 or younger on the day of the show)
- Men's Masters (40 or older on the day of the show)
- Women's Masters (35 or older on the day of the show)
- Men's Grand Masters (50 or older on the day of the show)
- Women's Grand Masters (45 or older on the day of the show)

The following are the male competitive classes. Some of these classes are divided even further, according to height and/or weight.

## Men's Physique

The men's physique division is aimed at men who prefer to develop a less muscular, yet athletic and aesthetically pleasing physique.

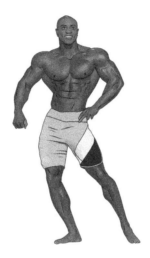

Men's physique classes range in height starting from physique A (Usually shorter than 5' 7") and typically going up to F (anyone over 6' 0").

Example:   Physique A - Up to and including 5' 7"
Physique B - Over 5' 7" up to and including 5' 8"
Physique C - Over 5' 8" up to and including 5' 9"
Physique D - Over 5' 9" up to and including 5' 11"
Physique E - Over 5' 11" up to and including 6'
Physique F - Over 6'

## Men's Classic Physique

Men's classic physique will be for competitors who want to present more muscular size than is currently acceptable for men's physique, but not as extreme as the current standards for bodybuilding.

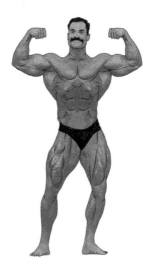

In order to qualify for the men's classic physique class, competitors are restricted to a particular height to weight ratio and are divided into divisions, just like men's physique.

Example: If a competitor is between 5' 6" and 5' 7" they can only weigh up to 175 lbs. Check your local federation for their specific guidelines.

## Men's Bodybuilding

Men's bodybuilding classes are for competitors who want to present a very muscular and developed physique. This is bodybuilding to the extreme.

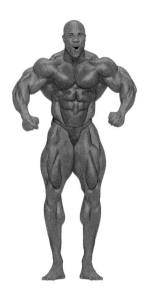

Men's bodybuilding is divided into weight classes only. There are no height restrictions. The general weight classes are as follows:

Example: Bantamweight - up to and including 143 lbs
Lightweight - up to and including 154 lbs
Middleweight - up to and including 176 lbs
Light-heavyweight - up to and including 198 lbs
Heavyweight - up to and including 220 lbs
Super heavyweight - over 220 lbs

The following are the female classes. Some of these classes are divided even further according to height and/or weight.

## Women's Bikini

Women's bikini competitors are very well toned with minimal visible muscle separation and even upper to lower body symmetry.

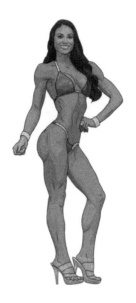

Bikini classes are divided into height classes, typically running from Bikini A to Bikini F.

Example: A - Up to and including 5' 1"
B - Over 5' 1" up to and including 5' 2.5"
C - Over 5' 2.5" up to including 5' 4"
D - Over 5' 4" up to and including 5' 5.5"
E - Over 5' 5.5" up to and including 5' 7"
F - Over 5' 7"

## Women's Wellness

Women's wellness division is similar to bikini except with larger shoulders, legs, and glutes creating a physique that is lower body dominant with slight separation and no striations.

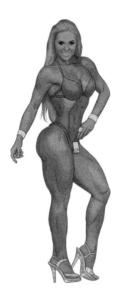

Wellness classes are divided into height classes, typically running from Wellness A to Wellness D.

Example:  Class A - Up to and including 5' 2"
Class B - Over 5' 2" up to and including 5' 4"
Class C - Over 5' 4" up to and including 5' 6"
Class D - Over 5' 6"

## Women's Figure

Women's figure is slightly more muscular than bikini, taking more of a Y shape, with slightly lower body fat percentages and modest muscle separation.

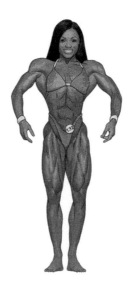

Figure classes are divided similarly to the bikini class, typically running from Figure A to Figure F.

Example:  A - Up to and including 5' 1"
B - Over 5' 1" up to and including 5' 2.5"
C - Over 5' 2.5" up to and including 5' 4"
D - Over 5' 4" up to and including 5' 5.5"
E - Over 5' 5.5" up to and including 5' 7"
F - Over 5' 7"

## Women's Physique

Women's physique classes are starting to venture more into the bodybuilding look, with a leaner physique and increased muscularity. Muscle separation and conditioning are becoming highlights in this class.

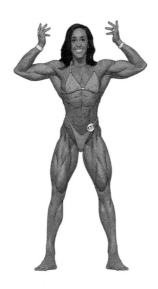

Women's physique class is generally divided into four classes, A to D.

Example:  A - Up to and including 5' 2"
B - Over 5' 2" and up to and including 5' 4"
C - Over 5' 4" and up to and including 5' 6"
D - Over 5' 6"

## Women's Bodybuilding

Like men's bodybuilding, the women's bodybuilding class is a physique that's taken to the extreme. Muscularity, conditioning, and muscle separation are huge factors in this class.

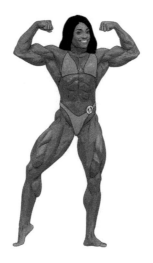

Women's bodybuilding is divided into weight classes. Height isn't a factor in this women's class.

Example:  Lightweight - Up to and including 115 lbs
Middleweight - Over 115 lbs up to and including 125 lbs
Light-heavyweight - Over 125 lbs up to and including 140 lbs
Heavyweight - Over 140 lbs

# Chapter 2:
# The Good

I will be the first one to admit that there are many positive aspects of the fitness industry that can easily be overlooked, not only by the general public, but also by the athletes within the industry itself. Most people will not succeed in meeting their goals because they keep focusing on the negative aspect of the industry instead of the positive. That shift in mindset can make or break a fitness career. Being competitive in the fitness world takes a ton of pain, planning, and effort.

I totally get it; sometimes it's really easy to fall into a discouraging mindset when almost every aspect of the sport is uncomfortable and difficult. Rest assured that the agony and discomfort that this sport brings is a blessing in disguise and this chapter is to remind people about the positive and beneficial aspects of bodybuilding.

## The New You

Fitness and bodybuilding is by far the best way to not only change one's physical body, but one's mindset as well. It gives people the ability to learn how to focus and concentrate. Every rep or activity can serve to push someone further physically and mentally than they ever had been before.

You will learn more about yourself when you are pushing to your utmost limitations during some sort of physical activity than you had in many years prior. This kind of stress is wonderful for personal growth. You will ask yourself questions such as, how determined am I? How much pain am I willing to endure to achieve my goal? Can I be consistent? Am I constantly willing to improve? Do I keep promises to myself? If I do screw up, am I willing learn from it, let it go, and keep moving forward? The list of questions can go on and on, but if you take a closer look, you can see how each of these questions can relate to life outside of fitness.

When people start their fitness journey, it's often because they want to change how they look. It's not always the case, but most of the time it is. My reason was because an ex-girlfriend cheated on me and I felt like I wasn't an attractive man anymore.

Changing one's body is something that is done to improve one's self-image. This change could be anything from losing weight, gaining weight, getting piercings or tattoos, to changing one's hair. As a result of change, a person can become more comfortable with themselves and therefore radiate their happiness and positive energy into the world.

There is no better feeling in the world than looking in the mirror, feeling comfortable in your own skin, and loving what you see. What most people don't realize is that you don't have to be "shredded" to be happy. Some people are happy being curvy, some love being ripped to the bone, some don't like having lots of muscles, and some do. All that matters is that you're happy when you look at yourself in the mirror. If you're not, well I have some good news for you—there are ways to change that. What better time to start than now?

When someone's fitness journey has started, it most definitely can be a love-hate relationship. The work is difficult, and it can push you to your mental and physical limits. This can be incredibly uncomfortable, but I promise you that when you walk out of that gym door, finish that run, or pack that kayak back into the truck, you will feel absolutely tremendous. All those endorphins and hormones running though the body after a workout gives you an astonishing natural high. Not only that, but recognizing that you've dominated a challenge for yourself will give you a massive boost in confidence. After a good workout, it's like some weight has been lifted off your shoulders and you see life in a whole new light.

This feeling increases at a phenomenal rate the harder you push yourself. After a few workouts, you really start to get a grasp on why fitness is so important to mental health. You start to learn how to respect your own body again. You begin to realize that this is the process of building the New You.

Since you're working so hard, you'll start to recognize that you don't want to waste all the hard work you're doing, so naturally, you start to make healthier life decisions. For example, you might reduce smoking, drinking, and eat a healthier diet.

A lot of the time people can fix chronic injuries or body issues they have been suffering with for years, such as inflexibility and joint problems. There are numerous documented cases of some types of diseases, such as diabetes, being reversed. The increase in natural endorphins and healthy hormones also increases the body's natural immune system, thus reducing the likelihood of minor illnesses such as the cold and flu. From personal experience, even if I do catch some sort of cold or flu, the effects are minimal compared to what they were like before I started living a healthy lifestyle.

When the body is allowed to return to running at an optimal level, miracles seem to happen. Skin, hair, and nails start to look healthier, and digestion starts to increase in efficiency. You have more energy and your emotions start to become more stabilized. Your metabolism increases, which means you can eat more food (healthy food) and have a slimmer waist. The density of muscle tissue increases, which raises the metabolism even more and helps reduce the risk of injuries, especially as one ages. Sleep improves, which has its own long list of benefits. You also start to enhance your stability and flexibility. This list can go on. Just imagine what that life would be like. A life of reduced illness, reduced likelihood of disease, a longer lifespan, etc. I don't know about you, but it seems like an easy choice to me.

Men and women obviously are very different from one another. The difference between men's and women's hormones and genetic makeup means the results each gets from body-building are going to be completely different, even if we train in a similar manner. I want to make things clear that if you are a woman and you lift weights, you are *not* going to start gaining massive amounts of muscle and start looking like a man. This is a myth. This just isn't going to happen, mainly because of the level of testosterone we all have in our bodies. It's no secret that men produce significantly more testosterone than women, which means men are naturally able to pack on significantly larger amounts of muscle and generally maintain a lower body fat percentage.

Women do not naturally produce enough testosterone to make these kinds of muscle gains. If you are a woman, the only way this will happen is if you genetically produce a lot of testosterone (which is rare), or if you are on some sort of anabolic steroid, which are modified versions of testosterone.

Will women gain some muscle lifting weights? Of course, but they won't be looking like a dude anytime soon. Ladies, please stop it with that ridiculous excuse for not picking up weights. You just need to do it. Gentlemen, this includes you too. How else are you going to bring your groceries into you house when you start aging? Walk up any stairs? Get up off the floor if you fall down? Get lifting those weights and start doing those damn squats. This is the New You we're talking about.

Lifting weights has also been proven to help increase bone density and reduce the risk of diseases such as osteoporosis for both men and women. Tendons (Attach muscle to bone) and ligaments (Attach bone to bone) attach to the surface of your bones. When muscle tissue increases in strength, your tendons and ligaments adapt as well. This allows them to allot more force onto the skeletal structure. Just like how muscles grow with stress, proper nutrition and training, bones can have the ability to strengthen as well. This can help to prevent 'bone erosion' aka Osteoporosis.

We all know how important sleep is for daily functioning. Sleep is essential for our physical and mental recovery. It can be difficult to get the sleep we need, because we live in a world that is moving faster and is more stressful than ever. Life in modern society has become frighteningly more demanding than in any other time in history. Unfortunately, many people sacrifice sleep in order to accomplish their daily tasks. We need our rest and we have to recognize that poor or insufficient sleep leads to slow and illogical decision making, emotional stress, physical and mental strain, less muscle recovery, decrease in life expectancy, slower reaction times, and more.

This is where fitness comes into play. After a workout, the body naturally puts itself into a state of relaxation. Your cortisol levels drop, and your serotonin levels start to skyrocket. This leads to an incredible increase in the quality of one's sleep.

We all know what it feels like to have an amazing night's rest. Waking up refreshed and ready for the day has its own list of benefits. Increased cognitive function, increased energy, better digestion, increased metabolism, reduced stress and inflammation, lower blood pressure and heart rate, increased physical and mental recovery are just a few things that are going to be life changing when you get enough sleep. Now imagine being able to get that quality of sleep on nightly basis. Fitness is an easy and healthy way to make this happen. Try it, I dare you. You'll thank me later.

Our lives are filled with distractions. When you start paying attention to how much you are being distracted, you'll be flabbergasted. Netflix, social media, cell phones, televisions, movies, etc., are time-sucking, life-wasting aspects in our lives. Most people don't even realize the huge amount of time they waste.

How about scrapping some of those distractions and using that time to get done what you need to during the day so you can get to bed on time and have a decent sleep? Here's a challenge: Start consciously recognizing how much of your time you waste during the day. I guarantee you'll be very surprised. Now use this time to be productive and change your life. Use that time to build the New You.

It can seem that people these days are working twice as hard just to get half of what previous generations had. The cost of living is rising, and there is no end in sight. People have less time to take care of their own personal needs as they work harder to make ends meet. This has led to processed foods becoming more and more of an acceptable dietary option in today's society.

Also, because people think they don't have time to eat healthy and are always on the go, they start to rely on stimulants to help keep them going throughout the day. Examples are coffee, tea, energy drinks, pre-workouts, fat burners, soda, ephedrine, etc.

Processed foods and stimulants are addictive, and it can be a little challenging to get off them. If you rely on stimulants, my advice to you is to slowly wean yourself off these things one at a time. Don't try to quit cold turkey. Trust me, in two days you're going to crash hard and be the grumpiest, most miserable person on the planet. Rather, wean down to two coffees a day, then start cleaning up your diet, one meal at a time. This can be a slow process but making slight changes will help tremendously with not only sleep, but overall health in general.

Honestly, living a healthy lifestyle isn't difficult. It only requires a little planning and execution. The basics of healthy living are eating a well-balanced, whole food diet, getting proper sleep, exercising, and consuming enough water. We all know this. The problem is people have this major disconnect with the execution. I don't know if it's just laziness, the lack of ambition, the fear of being uncomfortable, or even the fear of failure.

To execute healthy living, you just have to make it a priority and if you mess up, you mess up. Stop with the Netflix, stop being glued to social media, and stop watching TV for three or four hours a night. That's a massive amount of productive time wasted that could be used toward improving yourself. Use your time more effectively instead of wasting time on the couch. You could try prepping your meals for the next couple days, going to get some sort of exercises, reading a new book to improve cognitive function, or learning a new skill to help you in your professional or personal life.

In bodybuilding, hiring a good contest prep coach can be difficult at times. A contest prep coach is specialized in training clients to compete onstage. Asking around at a gym or searching Google is usually the best way to find a contest prep coach. You'll need to interview the coach before hiring them to make sure they are of good quality. We'll go into this later in this book with our interview with Ryan Richardson.

Transformation coaches, like myself, are a little easier to find. Do a quick Facebook search and you'll be able to find quite a few with relative ease. Transformation coaching is designed for clients looking to gain weight, lose weight, or maintain a certain body composition.

All coaches operate differently, and costs do fluctuate. Coaching has now generally moved online. This significantly reduces the cost for potential clients and gives the client more freedom to adapt their fitness journey to their daily schedules.

I recommend finding a coach that provides good quality communication, well balanced diets, and the ability to provide support when a fitness journey dips into a low. The ability to motivate and keep clients accountable is a sign of a good quality coach, whether they are a contest prep or transformation coach.

Consistency is the key to long-term success, in fitness and in life. We all know life can get in the way sometimes and we need to eat out or grab something that we shouldn't be eating. The important thing when this happens is to get right back on track and be as consistent as possible. We just need to learn from it, take the necessary steps to prevent it from happening again, and keep moving forward. There is no need to beat yourself up over it, just relax and realize you're human. Creating the New You is a process that takes time and practice.

Self-control needs to be trained just like a muscle. Think of it as a brain muscle that needs to be worked in order to grow. We are put into situations where we are invited to potluck dinners, lunch with the family, or wing night with friends. You can absolutely still go to these events. Nothing is stopping you from going, but this is the time where you get to practice flexing that self-control muscle. When all the food is around, practicing the ability to say no will be challenging at first. Basically, you're breaking the habit of saying yes, but if you can do it once, it gets easier every time after that. It will develop to the point where you won't even look at the bad food anymore. People will say, "Oh, just one bite won't hurt," or "Come on, it's Uncle's birthday," and try to guilt or convince you that it's okay. Just kindly let them know what you are trying to accomplish, and that eating that food does not help you accomplish your goal. Sometimes you will have to be a bit firmer with your response, but eventually they will get the point. If you do this a couple times, people won't even ask you anymore. The New You is more important than peer pressure trying to get in the way of your goals.

You will likely fail at this a time or two, but keep practicing. Just a warning though, taking just one bite will never just be one bite. Once your body gets a taste of that food you will want to have more. It's like a shark smelling the first drop of blood. It creates a food frenzy in your mind and you'll eat more without being able to stop yourself. Say no to the first bite and stick to that decision. You'll be extremely proud of yourself every time you do it.

People will start to comment on your self-control after you do this a time or two, and this will give you a massive boost in confidence. What I often do is bring pre-made meals with me to these events. That way I can still eat with everyone and feel like I'm part of the social gathering, and still stay on track with my meals while progressing to my goals. Invest in a meal prep bag. It's an adult-sized lunch box to always have your meal with you when you're on the go. They come in various sizes, shapes, and styles, so you have no excuse not to get one. My personal favourite is Six Pack Bags (www.sixpackbags.com). It's a great company with remarkable products. I highly recommend them as your meal prep bag option.

Sugar-free gum, diet soda, and soda water are also huge life savers. By the way, diet soda isn't water, so don't drink it like it is. Just drink it now and then to get you past cravings if you need to. I'll usually have a diet soda when I'm out at an event or social gathering. It helps quite a bit. Keep this in mind when you're at gatherings that have alcohol involved. People love trying to get other people to drink for some reason, but remember your goals. Do not stray off that path for anyone. It's not their life to live, it's yours.

Significantly reducing alcohol consumption is exceptionally important to living a successful healthy lifestyle for a couple of reasons. First, alcohol contains seven calories per gram. These calories are jam-packed with nothing but emptiness. They offer zero nutritional value whatsoever. Since the average drink contains about fourteen grams of alcohol, this means that the average beverage contains a minimum of ninety-eight calories. So, you can see how quickly these calories can add up. Even if you have just one drink a night every day of the week, that adds up to minimum of 686 calories per week and 2,744 added calories per month. When you remind yourself that it takes approximately 3,500 calories to burn off one pound of fat, you've just lost a significant amount of progress by having just one drink a day.

Two, alcohol slows down protein synthesis within the body at an exponential rate. Protein synthesis is one of the most fundamental processes in which the body rebuilds specific proteins. Without protein synthesis, we wouldn't be able to recover or heal.

What does this mean for you? This means that whenever you train or try to improve your body composition, your body won't have the ability to recover. This increases fatigue and significantly lengthens healing times, slowing your progress to a snail's pace. We know that the faster we heal and recover, the faster we can train again. The more we train, the greater the chance of hitting our fitness goals.

The last thing is to make sure you are getting enough water. Drink, drink, drink all day, every day. Yes, you are going to have to pee a lot until your body gets used to that amount of water, but don't make that an excuse to not drink it. We're talking about four litres (one gallon) a day minimum. I just heard some of you gasp reading that sentence. I do this every day; it's actually not that difficult. When I'm in peak week for a show, I'm water loading with upwards of eight to ten litres (two to two-and-a-half gallons) a day. Now that is a reason to gasp.

Hydration is a crucial component in fitness, and it provides a multitude of benefits for the body. We know that we are made up of over seventy percent water, so if we're dehydrated, we're turning ourselves into a raisin and raisins are gross. There is a reason they didn't name them dehydrated grapes like every other dehydrated fruit. If they did, no one would eat grapes anymore. Anyway, I got a little offtrack there.

Water is necessary for digestion, maximizing nutrient uptake and removing waste such as lactic acid and other toxic substances in the body. It also helps keep our blood pressure in a healthy range, keeps electrolytes balanced, and gives us the ability to sweat and cool ourselves off.

Water also plays a crucial role in strength. Just a three percent reduction in hydration (compared to body weight) can decrease muscular strength by up to nineteen percent. This is a massive drop. Water is also necessary to prevent cramping, fatigue, and decreased endurance. The moral of the story is that if you want to maximize your results, if you want the New You, stop crying about drinking that damn H2O. It's good for you.

A trick that I use to help get me into the right mindset about eating my meals and drinking my water is realizing how grateful I am to have access to all the resources necessary to get the results I want. We don't need to hike five miles a day through the desert just for two pails of water. We don't have to raise our own animals and slaughter our own meat. We have access to medical care, food, clothing, and world-class training facilities. We have roofs over our heads and food in our bellies.

If you want results and want to change how you feel about yourself, it literally couldn't be easier than it is now. Get off your butt, walk that twenty feet to the kitchen, turn on the tap, and waste that gallon of water just to get it ice cold before you drink it. Turn on that car or take that bus to get the food you need for the next week. If it's too cold to go to the gym, layer up. If it's too hot outside, drink some water and turn a fan on. We live in an extremely privileged world where *any* excuse is invalid. Give me an excuse and I guarantee you I will give you a solution. If you want the New You, a new life, or a new anything, stop making excuses and get it done.

All in all, this sport is just about making small, incremental steps to creating a better you. Any step forward helps. Drinking one more glass of water a day, eating out one day less a week, and walking for an extra fifteen minutes a day will help move you forward in creating the New You that you've always dreamed of. This goal isn't as far-fetched as you may think. With a little bit of thought and execution, the New You will soon be looking at you in the mirror.

# Community

Fitness and bodybuilding is a sport of community, connections, and friendships. If you stick with it long enough, you will develop lifelong relationships with people from all over the world. It doesn't take long for people to know who you are if you stay consistent. Being a positive, respectful, and personable human being in this industry is extremely important, especially if you plan on competing. Everyone loves a true sportsperson.

Bodybuilding isn't a sport that has a definitive winner like baseball or hockey. If you score a run or the puck hits the back of the net, you've scored a run or a goal. It's just that simple. It's not based on other people's opinions, it's purely definitive. Bodybuilding, however, isn't conclusive. When you compete, you are being judged by a panel of human beings. Although there are guidelines for judges to follow, these people still have slightly different opinions on what a competitor should look like and will subconsciously judge accordingly.

Although this can create some controversy, this is when sportsmanship plays a crucial role. If you lose, of course it's going to hurt, but you have to keep your composure and show integrity even if you think you should have won. That means no trash talking backstage, on social media, or to other people at the gym the next day. It is what it is and you can't do anything about it, so just move on.

This also works on the flip side. If you win, sure you're going to be ecstatic, and rightfully so, you just worked your ass off and came out on top. You deserve to be happy and excited, but realize that you won because the judges happened to like what you looked like on that particular day. It could have just as easily played into someone else favour. Be humble, respectful, and a true sportsperson. This is what people respect in this game, and in life in general. Remember that when you're training for a show, you're training to beat yourself, not other people. If you keep beating yourself, eventually you will win. This sport, and fitness in general, is a marathon, not a sprint.

Developing strong and positive relationships with people in the community is important in bodybuilding and fitness. These people help push you beyond your comfort level, help train you, and pull you out from the dark when you want to quit. These people basically live with you at the gym and compete against you at the shows. They become a second family with a common goal to help each other though the good times and the tough times. The relationships in this industry can be stronger than iron. Just like iron becomes stronger after it is exposed to high heat and cast into molds, so too are we molded by the iron we pump at the gym.

The community is tight. Respect is at the utmost importance if you want to succeed. The little group of people that you meet at the gym is the start of your own little community. It'll be your support system from inside, that truly knows the good, bad, and the heavy, so embrace it. The community you build around yourself can make or break your career.

You don't have to be a superstar to be known in this business. Over time, people will hear about you and recognize you from social media, contest pictures, or even just by hearing your name. This makes it important to be respectful everywhere you go. You will have a much better experience in this industry if you're a pleasant human being. We all know that there are assholes out there, and we tend to steer clear of those people because we don't want to be associated with them. Negativity, a poor attitude and/or image is unacceptable. You will enjoy a long, healthy career in bodybuilding and fitness for the rest of your life if you can stay grounded.

Once you get further into the sport and keep improving your physique, people will inevitably start complimenting you on how you look. Just accept these compliments. Some people have a hard time accepting them, and I'm one of those people. It takes some time to get used to, but it means you're making progress, and we all know progress is good news. Compliments make it easier to recognize that you're going in the right direction.

Social media plays a massive role in how we communicate, build relationships, and expand this sport. Support and new friendships are now just a click away. Our community just went from the people at the gym to everyone across the entire world in what seems to be a blink of an eye. It's growing faster than ever now that we're able to document our progress on the internet. If it wasn't for the internet, I truly believe that this sport would still be in the depths of the underworld. The internet has made it possible for the bodybuilding community to become larger than ever before and it is growing exponentially. Bodybuilding has been brought into a whole new light, where the general public gets to finally start to comprehend its true magnificence. We are still far behind in popularity than other mainstream sports, but bodybuilding will eventually get there. Thank you, social media, and thank you, internet.

Side note, if you want to be part of the fitness and bodybuilding community, here's another little fact that bodybuilders have to deal with. Moving people's stuff. People will always want you to help them move. Just accept this fact. It's going to happen all the time. Just make sure there's pizza involved to make up for the unscheduled calorie deficit. Add pineapples to that Italian pie too and screw what other people think about it.

# A Sport for Everyone

This sport is not bound by age, ability, race, gender, or anything in between. Every single person on this planet can benefit from fitness in one way or another. You don't need to be an extrovert to enjoy it. Introverts, like myself, can also enjoy training, because once you get changed, throw on your headphones and blare your tunes, you enter your own world.

The gym is a place of self-improvement; a place where people can go to improve their mood, vision, self-esteem, and attitude. Some people, like myself, use fitness and bodybuilding as a way to meditate, and without it we would be lost. Others use it as a way to stay healthy, get out of the house, or to bond with friends and family. Some take things to the next level and start bodybuilding for a living. Everyone and anyone can enjoy health, fitness and bodybuilding no matter what level they want to take it too.

Just like every other sport, genetics plays a huge role in someone's success in bodybuilding. Some things about your body you just can't change. For example, your muscle and skeletal structures. Do you have small or large muscle bellies? How well does your body put on muscle? How wide are your shoulders? How slim is your waist? Do you have small or large joints? Do you have long bones or short bones in relation to your height?

All these things play a role in how successful you will be in the sport, and only a select few will have the opportunity to become a champion. Yes, dedication, talent, and hard work will absolutely help if someone lacks some genetic privileges, but if someone with genetics more suited to bodybuilding works just as hard, 99.99 percent of the time they will win the competition.

I don't want to ruin anyone's day, but you have to be honest with yourself if you decide to take competing seriously. This is for both men and women, and competing is literally going to change every aspect of your life. So, ask yourself if you actually have a body type that could truly compete in bodybuilding. Most people don't, but they still try (Good for them for trying, though!) and end up heartbroken and devastated when they can't win or place at a show over and over again.

But here is the good news: social media has instantly changed how successful a bodybuilder can be. Bodybuilders don't need to win a single competition to become famous or successful these days. Genetics doesn't even play a role in the success outside of competitions anymore. As a result, it has levelled the playing field for aspiring bodybuilders all over the world, no matter how talented or genetically privileged they may or may not be.

For example, there are people who have millions of followers on Instagram just because they have a nice ass. They literally take pictures of their ass all day and get paid for it. What the hell am I doing wrong here? I thought my ass was finer than a fine wine. Apparently not.

Although competing in this sport may not be for everyone, the sport itself is. Yes, there is a difference between the two. For example, I'm not going to be passing pucks to Sidney Crosby in an NHL game anytime soon, but I still enjoy going to the pond in the winter and shooting some pucks around.

It doesn't matter who you are or what you do, you can enjoy this sport. It will keep you healthy, moving, and living a longer, happier life. I know people in their young teens and people into their late years who thoroughly enjoy bodybuilding and fitness. Everyone from doctors, lawyers, tradespeople, first responders, retail employees, students, people with any type of disability, and everyone in between are enjoying this sport. I've met them, I've competed beside them, and I've trained them. What's your excuse? If you think bodybuilding or fitness isn't for you, you are thoroughly mistaken.

# Chapter 3:
# The Bad

Like any other sport, there is a darker side to bodybuilding. Every sport has something that can put a significant strain on the body. There is a reason professional athletes get paid the big bucks. They are literally putting their health, mind, and body at significant risk every single day. Professional bodybuilding is no different. We are exposed to all sorts of obstacles, not only potential harm to the body. It can go much deeper than that.

## Groundhog Day

The words "Groundhog Day" in the realm of bodybuilding don't even do it justice. It is literally the same thing over and over and over again. Sleep, eat, train, eat, work, eat, eat, go home, eat, sleep, and repeat. When I said this sport is scheduled and regimented, I wasn't joking. Sometimes you will even get your days confused. "Is it Sunday or Wednesday? I have no idea."

You had better get used to living the same day over and over again, because that consistency is how people succeed in this sport. It will get overwhelming and exhausting at times. You will debate many times whether or not this is the path you really want to go down. Some people get to the point where they start to think that they've wasted all their life being in the gym for hours on end every day. Perhaps they could have lived a more exciting and joyful life. To be honest, it's probably true. I even wonder about those same things sometimes. I think, why am I doing this with my life? Where is this going to take me? Is it really worth all the sacrifices such as my time, friends, family, and health? Would it not have been better to just pursue the fire department, have a great career with a decent salary, benefits, and the opportunity to take regular vacations? My wallet would be much thicker if I wasn't in this sport; I could have probably owned a house or two by now. Is it worth it?

It's going to be extremely tough mentally. If you do one or two shows, sure, it's not going to be that bad. You will still be asking yourself some of these questions at some points throughout the process, though. If you're wanting to do this for a living, you need to be mentally ready to immediately dismiss these thoughts as they creep up.

There is something about doing the same thing over and over again that can wear some people down to the point of hatred and disdain. Personally, I tend to feed off this regimented scheduling. I know what my daily tasks are and I know what I'm expecting each day. It works for me. Sure, I still have some bad days, but I'm mainly in my comfort zone. For a lot of other people though, it's not. They can only take it for so long before they crack. You have to know yourself. Can you deal with this kind of repetitive lifestyle?

There are some ways to mix things up. One way is to change the times you train. This is good shock to the system, too. Not only will you feel like your schedule is different, your body will also be shocked by this change. If your body is used to training after work at 5:30 p.m. every day for three months, then when you start training at 6:00 a.m. before work, your body is going to be like "What the fuck are you doing, man? This isn't right" and it'll have to adapt to the new time. To a degree, even this slight but sudden change can be enough to help break though plateaus and get your body responding again.

Another small change is training in a different gym or training with a different partner. Some gyms have different equipment, which means you'll be able to work the same muscle groups in a slightly unfamiliar manner. This is also a great shock to the body, and what do we know about shocking the body? It means growth and progress.

Also, every gym has a different atmosphere. It could even just be a different location of a gym you already have a membership to, but still, the atmosphere will be different. Some people like to debate me on this, but even a mental shock like a change in gym atmosphere is great for muscle gains. It can get you into a different headspace to train harder. There are no distractions at a new gym, no one you know to talk to, and nothing but focused work. This is the perfect headspace to be in when training.

Another Groundhog Day experience you're going to encounter is that of eating your meals. After about three days of dieting, you're going to heat up a meal and before you even take your first bite you're going to say, "Again? This shit again?" I was literally laughing when I wrote this last sentence, because I just said that about ten minutes ago when I was eating my last meal. I literally said to myself, "Damn it, here we go again." This will never end, but after I do my half second of complaining, I tell myself, "I'm eating for a purpose, for a goal, and not for flavour. Stop being a baby and eat it." Then I eat it, and I'm good until the next meal when I'll have the same discussion with myself.

Getting through the endless repetitiveness of this life is about recognizing your small wins. It makes life so much more enjoyable in this sport. I literally celebrate every meal I eat.

I pat myself on the back and say, "One more meal closer to my dream. BOOM!" and I drop my fork like a hot mic. I get my training done and I'm like, "Another back day closer to having the best back in the industry. BOOM!" and I drop my headphones into my bag like another hot mic. I'm basically dropping hot mics all day. It's great. I love it.

Don't be afraid to celebrate your small victories. It could be anything, such as getting out of bed early to work out because you can't at any other time during the day, or not turning on your TV and using that time to do meal prep instead, or consuming all your meals that day, or drinking all your water that day. Any small win will help motivate and distract you from the monotony of everyday life in bodybuilding. Plus, those small celebrations always lead to bigger ones. So, keep dropping them mics no matter how small the victory.

Just like anything, if you do the same thing over and over again or eat the same thing over and over again, you're going to get sick of it. Making just the smallest adjustment can help break that cycle. Train at a different time, use a different spice when seasoning your food, eat different proteins, mix up your carbs, train at a different gym, or train with a different training partner. All these things can help you get though the wearisome nature of this sport.

# Personal Relationships

**This section's special guests are Alfred and his wife Shauna Voit. Alfred is an IFBB pro with a champion of a wife that has been by his side throughout his entire journey. Their perspective on maintaining a healthy relationship while living the life of bodybuilding is invaluable. (Instagram: @ alfredvphysique_ifbb_pro and @shaunavoit)**

This section is filled with emotions, facts, and some information that, for some people, may be hard to comprehend, but it's necessary.

Everyone deserves a chance to live a life with someone they love. The last thing I want is someone losing the love of their life to this sport when all that was needed was a little perspective, communication, and an understanding of what it takes for a relationship to survive the hardships of the fitness and bodybuilding industry.

When you get deeper into this industry, you will soon realize that this kind of life isn't designed for people that aren't personally involved with it. You will notice that most people that are a part of the fitness and bodybuilding industry are single, or, in most cases, have a partner that is involved with the sport as well.

Involving yourself in a relationship with someone that is living the bodybuilding and fitness life helps immensely. They understand the process and the extents you have to put yourself through to achieve your goals. They understand that training isn't an option and it must be done. They understand that you need to stay on point with your diet and that your recovery is crucial. They also understand when you're grumpy. That's because being "hangry" (hungry + angry = hangry) is almost a permanent emotional state during the last weeks of a contest prep. You both get to help and support each other through the hard times in this sport. If both parties know how it feels, everyone is much more understanding of the processes involved.

Unfortunately, dating someone outside the fitness world rarely ends up being successful. Through the years of watching this sport chew up and spit out relationships like it's bubble gum (including some of my own), I have recognized that dating outside the sport usually means a doomed relationship.

I'm not saying it's impossible for a relationship with someone outside the sport to work, it just takes a tremendous amount of effort to keep the relationship healthy and thriving. There are relationships that last though the stress, but they do have their own bundle of challenges.

When you get deep into competing, everything needs to be on point. There is zero room for error. This inevitably means that sacrifices will have to be made. The most common sacrifice is time. Time with your family and friends. This is where most issues stem from when being in a relationship with a competitive bodybuilder or fitness enthusiast. Meals need to be eaten on time, training needs to be done every day, rest and recovery is essential and food prep must be done to maximize the chances for success. There are no ifs, ands, or buts about it. This is just fact, so when anything gets in the way of contest prep, it can become a major issue.

Bodybuilding is a very selfish sport. In your mind you're going to think, "I can't sacrifice my success for a movie/dinner/evening out, etc. I'm working too hard to risk losing my show because of this." This is exactly where a lot of the issues in relationships with bodybuilders or fitness enthusiasts begin. This attitude makes it look like all you care about is bodybuilding, and this is exactly why this sport is indeed a selfish one. You need to get what you need done first before you can enjoy other life activities, but by the time you finish these essential tasks of contest prep, the day is usually over. The saying "work before play" is real with this sport, because most times it seems like it's ninety-nine percent work and one percent play. This can make a partner feel unwanted and unloved. Trust me, it's a very tricky balance to have a personal relationship and a bodybuilding lifestyle. Everything revolves around you and how you can adjust your schedule for the greatest chance of success.

Last-minute plans won't work, they just don't. If plans come up last minute and I still have training and food prep to do, I'm sorry, but I can't do it. This is my career at stake, and I can't let anything get in the way of that, and my wife understands. It also works the other way around. If she is preparing for a show, I would never let anything get in the way of her success. This means that if she or I need to attend a gathering alone, then that's exactly what's going to happen. The last thing we want to do is to put each other's success at risk. Mutual understanding and patience in our relationship is extremely important.

The best way to achieve this, whether you're in a relationship with a competitor or not, is to try to plan your weeks in advance. This has been a very helpful strategy in my personal relationship, making it possible to properly prepare for future events without having to sacrifice our goals.

Having a strategy makes your personal life a little bit easier to deal with. It is going to take a little effort to figure it out, and you're probably going to have a fight or two about this, but it is possible to be in a relationship with someone when you're in this sport. It will take a lot of communication, an understanding of the bigger picture and your goals, and patience. Lots and lots of patience.

**Shauna** - *"I did my best to help him where I could when he did his preps, but really he just let me do it my way, let me shop, let me do my thing, and that was fine and I think I generally gave him the space to do what he needed to do and I took care of other stuff so he wouldn't have to worry about it. Then year two, two and a half and he's doing another show. It starts to affect our old friendships that were couples. There were mutual friends that we had together and slowly he was starting to just get into the competitions. Which meant meeting a lot of single people, young people, and I* *wasn't really a part of it right, except from seeing the shows. So, I started to think, 'okay, are you changing or what's going on?' I started to feel isolated and I'd say, 'You know, this is getting lonely. I don't have my partner here."*

**Alfred** - *"Still to this day it's tough."*

**Shauna** - *"Part of my problem is I hold things and I may say things sarcastically and spitefully, but I think I would let things sort of sit with me and then they get in my head. Days pass, you can see something brewing. It could just be the smallest thing, but it's that one thing where I'm just ignited. We'll have our moment and then a few days later when we're both calmer I'll say, 'Look, I understand you're this type of personality, you need these outside things in your life, but you've got to understand where I'm coming from and see it from a different point of view that when you do these things this is how it's making me feel". He's always very good at that point. First, we're all defensive, but at that point he's very good. He goes away, thinks about it, comes back and makes adjustments. If he wasn't like that, we wouldn't have been able to go forward. So I do think it's about communication, talking and both being willing to commit to a different level of the relationship."*

You have to remember you have other people to think about, too, such as your partner, friends, and family. You can see how having a personal life as a bodybuilder can be extraordinarily difficult. You're probably going to lose friends, it's almost guaranteed if bodybuilding is what you want to do with your life. I have lost many friends to this sport and I assure you, they probably won't be the last ones. Since this is a 24/7 sport, anyone in your life that is outside the industry usually ends up being pushed out. This doesn't necessarily mean that these people are gone completely or forever. This just means that you'll likely not be seeing them or hanging out with them as often. Sometimes yes, they will leave, and you will never see them again. Friends come and go; it's normal, so don't beat yourself up over it. It's just a part of life.

Family, on the other hand, is a little bit trickier to deal with. Of course, they're your family and they will always love you and want the best for you, but there is something about this sport that most family members don't understand. Like the amount of time it requires. You will find family members disappointed in you for missing a dinner or not being able to see them on a regular basis. Some might be furious. It happens, but what's important is you need to communicate to them that this is your life. This sport requires sacrifices and you're happy doing it. Happiness should be the first thing your family wants for you anyway, so if you're truly happy becoming a bodybuilder, then they should be happy for you.

Sometimes family just won't let it go. They won't get off your ass about the sport you love, and all you hear from them is negativity, disappointment, and bullshit after more bullshit. I'm not saying this should be done without consideration, but if they aren't going to support you, maybe it's time to let that person go, too. You need to surround yourself with positivity and promise. With encouragement and assurance, not negativity and nagging. This business is hard enough as it is, and the last thing you need is that kind of attitude from your own family.

If you want to be a champion, you need to start surrounding yourself with champion-like people. The "Sum of Five" rule indicates that you are the average sum of the five people you hang out with the most. Meaning, if the five closest people to you make thirty-five thousand dollars a year, you're likely only going to be making thirty-five thousand dollars a year. If you're forty pounds overweight, the five people closest to you are likely to be an average of forty pounds overweight as well. This concept applies to basically everything in life and it doesn't seem to make an exception for bodybuilding.

# Social Media

Social media is driving the growth of the bodybuilding industry at a tremendous rate. This means the potential for high-dollar contracts, sponsorships, and Hollywood-like attention is about to start becoming a serious reality.

For most amateur athletes, though (and even for most pros), this requires a ton of work to keep their presence known on social media. The second their social media presence dies down, they basically fall into the dark abyss of other up-and-coming athletes. It's up to the athletes themselves to consistently market themselves on as many relevant platforms as possible. This is a full-time job on its own.

Now imagine you're a spouse of a bodybuilding athlete, observing that their attention is constantly on social media at work, at home, on dates, at the dinner table, etc. Now imagine them following, conversing, and building relationships with people with some of the best-looking physiques in the world. It doesn't take a genius to realize that this is probably going to be an issue.

**Alfred** - *"One of the biggest problems in the relationship with being in the fitness industry for me was social media. It's huge, and it's a problem today. It's a problem right now because I'm dying to pick that up right now to check."* (*Pointing at his phone.*)

**Shauna** - *"I say to him all the time that social media will kill a marriage unless you start being more aware of it."*

Social media is a huge driving force of the sport. Everyone wants to get sponsored; everyone wants to get noticed and involved. The only time it doesn't matter is when people don't want to continue anymore.

When you become an IFBB pro, there is an expectation of maintaining social media presence, and you almost become a slave to social media. People want to know what you're up to, they want to be encouraged by you, motivated by you, you want to feel like your pro card means something and that you're giving back.

**Shauna** - *"Sometimes with the social media I'm sitting here and he's sitting there for forty-five minutes on his phone. Sometimes you feel lonelier when you're with someone than if you were just on your own. Like during the day I can be on my own doing whatever and I don't feel lonely. Then he comes into the house and all of a sudden I feel very alone because we're not connecting. That bond's not there."*

**Alfred** - *"There's always something that comes up and I'm on my phone too much when she's around. Now I try to think, 'Okay she's here, click, shut it off and she's like, 'You don't need to go off your phone just because I step into the room.' I'm like, 'I'm doing it out of respect' and she goes, 'I know you're thinking about it.' And I'm like, 'You know what, can I not do anything right here?'"*

**Shauna** - *"I'm not feeling connected with him because he's sitting on his frickin' phone connecting with all these other people. And I'm like, 'Okay, a majority of the people you* are following are frickin' bikini girls. I'm sitting here soft as ever and you're going through this feed and of course it's all tits and ass and everything else.' I'm starting to think that he's coming to bed with these pictures of what he's just been scrolling though. So, it's like, when are we going to get a break from this?"

**Alfred** - "*There's still challenges, but it's definitely gotten a lot better. And also with social media, you get random people just sending you message, hearts, and sending you certain types of messages.*"

**Shauna** - "*I understand the social media. You put stuff out there and you can't control what people are putting back, but there was a degree to which I was starting to see that Alfred was engaging.*"

**Alfred** - "*It was to encourage other people, but it would come across sometimes as ...*"

**Shauna** - "*Yes, he's doing it for the likes, he's doing it for the engaging, he's doing it for this. From my point of view, it looks like my husband is sitting here engaging and blowing kisses and heart eyes and 'you're a real smoke show' and 'no filters needed for this.' It's like, I'm supposed to be your babe. This is getting to a point now where it's too much.*"

**Alfred** - "*Yeah, it's a stupid concept and that's not my personality. I don't go up to someone and say, 'Oh you're a bombshell.' I just don't do that because I'm respectful to people. That's where I needed to regulate and say okay, enough with the comments and stuff like that.*"

It is clear from Alfred and Shauna's comments that regulating time on social media is an extremely important skill that must be learned to make a relationship with a fitness professional a successful one.

There will be bumps in the road while learning how to manage social media time appropriately, but what's important is the constant communication and making adjustments so neither party feels unloved or unwanted.

The fitness lifestyle is completely different from the average human lifestyle. The people, the environment, and attitude etc. is all different. When you're in a relationship with someone who isn't as much a part of this world as you are, it can feel like you're living two completely different lives. You have the fitness life and a life back home.

**Alfred** - *"I could still come home and have my family life and everything like that, but then all the bodybuilding, physique competitions, interacting with those types of people, it was another world."*

**Shauna** - *"He's doing all these fun things, going out and he's not even asking me 'cause he's like, 'Well, I didn't think you would want to.' I was like, 'How am I supposed to appreciate what you're getting into if I'm not even going to be brought into it,' right?' I don't know if he even really wanted me to, deep down. I think he was just enjoying being so ..."*

**Alfred** - *"Well, you get so much attention. When you're doing well, I mean, it's an amazing feeling and you're kind of on your own. You feel like you're on your own and it's a surreal lifestyle."*

**Shauna** - *"I think he was starting to enjoy separating it."*

Unfortunately, fitness and bodybuilding is littered with infidelity. It doesn't help that it's a singles-dominated industry.

During a competition, there are a couple hundred competitors (men and women) that are looking the best they ever have. They're tanned, they're all done up with makeup, they're wearing tight stage bikinis and posing trunks. After the show is over, they celebrate their victories and losses with some food and drinks. You now have a town full of people loosened up with drinks and their confidence is through the roof. You have guys on steroids that are ready to bang a hole in the wall with hundreds of good-looking women that are usually staying at the same hotel. This is a recipe for infidelity if I ever saw it, and unfortunately it happens quite a bit.

> **Shauna** - *"It is an environment that is mostly singles, because a lot of them [relationships] don't work because of a lot of this I think. People don't understand the commitment and the focus, and it doesn't work. Like you were saying, you've been in relationships with people that weren't in competitions and they don't understand what's involved."*

> **Alfred** - *"It would be back and forth because she would explain how she felt and I would try to put her at ease, saying, 'You know that I'm not going out with these girls, I'm not doing what you think I'm doing.'"*

> **Shauna** - *"don't want to give too much information, but he's all geared up here. He's fired to go like every five minutes and I'm feeling like we have zero connection here right now. You're on Instagram, engaging with whoever and you're out with whoever. You come home and I see you for an hour after training and you wanna like, get on here, and I'm sitting here like, yeeaahh."*

**Alfred** - *"Guys were always going after her when we were younger and I was always chasing down these dudes like, 'Get the fuck away from my girl!' Now all of a sudden, I'm getting all this attention and it was tough for me to take. Not tough, it was enjoyable, but I don't know, I didn't know how to deal with it. I mean, when I was younger, I thought I was okay-looking and stuff and girls would come up to me but, oh my god, this was just crazy once you're in this industry."*

**Shauna** - *"As much as you trust and you have loyalty, shit happens, and in this industry, there are people that are barking up who-evers tree. There are women there if he (Alfred) has is wedding ring on, it's more of a challenge. Like they don't care, and when he's not making me a priority it's even more of a temptation. This is an industry that's rampant with infidelity and open relationships. I just wanted him to not look at me like, 'You're being jealous, you're being crazy, you're being insecure, you're being needy.' I just wanted him to say, 'I get what you're saying,' and reassure me that he could see it and understand. I probably would have settled down a lot more if he had given me that."*

It's very difficult to see your significant other in an industry full of extremely good-looking people when you're not fully involved in the industry yourself. I completely understand that feeling. I met my wife six weeks before a competition. The competition was out of town and I asked her not to attend. Not only did I ask her not to come, but I would also be staying in the same hotel as my ex whom I had broken up with a few weeks prior to meeting my wife.

My girlfriend (now my wife), understandably, wasn't very impressed. We fought about it, and resolved the issue. Obviously, she thought I was going to be up to some scandalous shit, but actually, I didn't want to take the chance of looking like a loser in front of her if things went sideways at the competition. I didn't want her to see me as a losing bodybuilder she's now dating. I came in second in that competition, so my fear was clearly blown out of proportion.

There is some sort of relationship drama with people at almost every competition. Someone's barking up the wrong tree or people barked up a tree together that they shouldn't have. I swear, sometimes it's like high school all over again.

For that reason, I like to stick to myself. I like to stay in the shadows as much as possible, show up to compete, and retreat right back into the shadows. It keeps me sane and keeps my relationships intact. That's how I deal with it. Others will find their own way. Some people like the attention and the glory and will have to deal with the repercussions that it brings.

It's important to have your significant other involved and in the loop. Open communication is what kept Shauna and Alfred's relationship alive and flourishing. Whether your spouse is in the sport or not, communicate. With communication, it doesn't matter how choppy the water gets, the boat can stay afloat.

A few days after interviewing Alfred and Shauna, Shauna sent me an excellent email containing some amazing insights on what they did to adapt their relationship to get through life with Alfred being an IFBB Pro. The following is what I received:

> "As Alfred said, we still have challenges with it all, and social media and disconnect is a big challenge. However, it comes down to how much one values and respects the relationship and the other person. How important is it to you? A serious athlete understands more than anyone what it means to be committed, focused, and mentally and physically present. In my opinion, the only way it works and remains healthy

and loving is when egos are set aside. Only then can true communication be at the forefront and you really hear each other. Treat each other the way you want to be treated. Alfred and I agreed that being an athlete should require being professional. If the athlete approaches their goals and interactions in a professional manner, it will provide respect and boundaries. Not only set the athlete up going forward, but also protect their relationship. Alfred did this by stepping back, being more mindful with his interactions through social media and in the circuit. There are many layers of superficial aspects, so taking time to reflect and ask, how is this serving me and those I care about? Keeps things real and aligned. Every once in a while, an athlete needs a gentle reminder and reigning in. The other partner also has to be willing to be part of the lifestyle. Training together, clean eating together, being open to the culture and sharing in the events together. Recognizing how important and fulfilling it is to them and then provide that support from a loving place. Whatever works to make it shared and inclusive. That said, a huge part of making this work for us is when the athlete stops and recognizes that through all of their dedication, training, hard work, time and financial investment, it has meant that their partner has made sacrifices for them. Giving up social gatherings, holidays, personal goals, whatever it may be ... sacrifices have been made for them. It had a big impact when Alfred acknowledged this on a deeper level, and it made me feel valued that he finally understood where I was coming from. Now he tries to find ways to honour me in our relationship.

When this is done regularly and consistently (daily) we are in a very good place, and support is being reciprocated. This was a big one, I feel it was key for Alfred and I."

# Costs

**This section's special guest is Karen Harrison. She has not only been an ER nurse for more than twenty years, but she is also my mother. In my opinion, she is the best source of information, from a family member's viewpoint, on what it is like to be close to but not involved in the industry.**

Bodybuilding is an expensive sport. The expenses seem to increase the deeper one digs down into the bodybuilding rabbit hole. Costs include hiring a coach and a nutritionist, registration costs, suits, travel, accommodations, supplements, gym memberships, recovery treatments (chiropractors, massage therapy, acupuncture, etc.), tanning, hair and makeup, food, jewelry, tickets for friends and family to watch you, and for some people, the costs of anabolic steroids. You can see how these things can quickly add up.

> **Karen** - *"The expense! My son needed to eat a lot, and good, clean food is so much more expensive. Food is expensive, and it's a terrible thing that eating like crap costs less money but fills the tank. It was always something a single mom had to deal with every day. Then you have all your supplements and vitamins etc. Money is always a friend and a nemesis!"*

If I were to compete again at a small, local, non-tested regional show, it would cost me between three and five thousand dollars. This is just a regional show. Now imagine if you have to travel across the country or even to a different country to compete. How about competing more than once a year? You can see that these costs can skyrocket. You have to be ready for this.

I know many people, including myself, that have two jobs just to feed the hungry money machine of this sport. For me, I know this is going to be my life. I absolutely love it, therefore I don't care that I've had to work two jobs to afford it. Some people work three or four jobs. We do what we have to, to do what we love. This is the kind of commitment it takes to compete on a regular basis.

If you're in a relationship or have a family, a conversation about the financial commitment required for this sport is crucial. Everyone needs to be ready. Remember, failing to prepare is preparing to fail and that includes situations like this. Everyone needs to be on the same page, because the cost isn't only monetary. It costs your time (a lot of it), your emotional state, and for some people, their health.

**Karen** - *"It was hard not seeing my son. That kind of blindsided me, going from seeing him all the time to barely at all. Honestly, I thought it was because he didn't want to see me. I always felt I was not the best mom, and that was the reason for him to be away from home. It was also hard seeing how it affected his relationship with Dana, the mother of his child. It did seem that he was leaving Dana and Harley, his daughter, a lot more than he did before, and I was worried about his relationship with both of them. I know it really affected Dana, and I felt for her, being left alone so much. I felt for my son too. I worried about how he was feeling, and wishing I knew how to fix things. Looking back, neither of us really understood it. I did know that he was very focused on it and I could not stand in his way. I just had to be there for him if things went sideways."*

The sport of bodybuilding can be very difficult for family to be involved in. In order to see a loved one compete, you must purchase tickets to watch the show. Most shows are set up with a morning show (where the competitors are compared and prejudged) and an evening show (where the judging is confirmed and the awards are given out). This is a double whammy, because tickets are not only horrendously overpriced, now you have to buy a ticket to each show if you want to see your loved one compete and possibly receive an award.

A ticket to each show can run upwards of seventy-five to one hundred twenty-five dollars. No one should be paying these kinds of prices. In my opinion, this is exponentially holding back this sport from its true potential. For this reason, I refuse to have my family come to my shows. I will not let them spend that kind of money just to see me onstage for a few minutes.

**Karen** - *"Not being able to see my son compete makes me sad. It is just too expensive when you have to pay two hundred dollars for the day. It's a shame, really. Maybe if it wasn't so expensive, more people would come to the shows."*

Not only are the financial costs of bodybuilding high, but so are the physical and mental costs. There is no other sport on this planet that requires you to deplete the body to the extreme while still having to maintain the highest level of performance. Imagine if a hockey player had to deplete their body to the extreme but still have to maintain performance, or how about a football or baseball player. I'm not saying these sports don't take skill, because they absolutely do, and these professionals are incredibly talented. They are the best in the world, but let's compare darts to hockey.

Unlike any other sport, bodybuilding is a 24/7 sport. If you're serious, there is no off-season. You're constantly on a diet and your weight and cardiovascular training never ends.

**Karen** - *"I think my advice to those going into it is this: doing this takes discipline and sacrifice, such as friends and family time, so think about it and make sure you can deal with the negative effects. Tell those who love you what it is* *and why you're doing it. It wasn't until Chris talked to me and told me about it and what he wanted out of it that I started to understand it and not take him being away so personally. The expense to do it right and the time it will take also needs to be considered. Have a plan."*

# Politics

Politics is a very real issue in bodybuilding. Just a one-off comment on social media, or to someone you know about a judge or another competitor can come full circle and bite you. Word travels fast in the bodybuilding and fitness world. It only takes a second for things to get blown out of proportion.

If you're an a-hole off the stage, you're probably not going to win a meaningful show. These federations want winners that respect the industry. They want people that are going to reflect a positive image of the sport and the federation to help them both grow. So, if you think that being tough and talking trash and disrespecting people is the way you're going to get to the top, you're going to be in for a big surprise.

Some panel judges are now adding and creeping athletes on social media. They are getting an idea of who you are outside of the gym. Are they supposed to? That's a grey area. Although the judges shouldn't take into consideration an athlete's life outside the stage, when they are judging the physiques at a show, they subconsciously will.

If you're a prick off the stage and they hear about it from another person or they see it on social media, when you walk onstage that's the very first thing they are going to think about. They'll be like, "Oh this person was such an a-hole a couple months ago. Their sportsmanship isn't what we're looking for," and boom, now the judges are likely to subconsciously score lower. This does happen, and it makes perfect sense.

Sportsmanship is extremely important. It symbolizes professionalism and respect, which are some of the most valuable factors this sport needs in order to flourish. If you're not professional, or a good sportsperson, you can forget about your chances of winning a competition. Your energy is better spent by focusing on positivity and training.

Politics don't start and end with talking trash and having a negative attitude. Sometimes things like possible future placings, popularity, and marketability can play a role in how judges look at you. I bet you're thinking this doesn't make any sense in a sport that's all about physiques. Well, that's because it doesn't. This is another major downfall of this industry. At the end of the day, this is a form of entertainment. The industry is trying to attract people in as many ways as possible. If that means letting someone win who is more popular to increase the federation's reach, then that's exactly what's going to happen.

Obviously, the quality of the physiques between first and second has to be very close to get away with this kind of move. Although this doesn't seem to be happening as often anymore, It does happen, so I suggest you start marketing yourself as much as you can as early as possible.

Brand yourself uniquely and set yourself apart compared to anyone else. Just to show the real you in your social media. Be vulnerable and open; people respect openness and honesty. This will get your audience to know you, trust you, and like you. This little secret will make your social media explode and make you unique from everyone else in the industry.

Here is another little secret: Not everyone is going to like you. This is a tight community, which means some people think they need to be friends and liked by everyone, but this isn't the case. Some people won't like you. It happens in the sport and it happens in life. The best course of action is to just be mature and stay out of each other's hair.

Who you hang out with and the reputation of the people closest to you can play a role in your placings. For example, if you hang out and spend most of your time with people that have the reputation of being a-holes, people are going to associate you with that kind of reputation whether you're an a-hole or not. It's not fair, but unfortunately that is just how the world works. Why would judges place an athlete who has the potential to involve poor quality people in the industry? I wouldn't, especially if I were trying to grow a professional bodybuilding federation.

Other major professional sports organizations do background checks on athletes that they want to sign. If the professional code of conduct around an athlete's personal life isn't up to par, they likely won't get signed. The organization won't risk that kind of negative attention. Sure, sometimes people slip through the cracks, but there is most definitely a screening process in professional sports.

Bodybuilding is trying to become a highly paid mainstream sport, so if you want to get ahead, I suggest being on the straight and narrow. If you're not, start hanging out with some good quality influences immediately, and turn away from the ones who will not serve your future.

Remember that politics are present in social media as well. Social media can be an amazing tool to use to your advantage but time and time again I have seen social media crush people's reputation and career just as fast as they built it. Becoming a social media influencer seems to affect some people's ability to lose focus on reality. Loyalty to sponsors and brands that have supported athletes are dropped to the highest bidder or to the company that provides the most free product. Once that well dries up, they're onto the next sponsor. It only takes a couple of moves to different brands for people to realize your lack of loyalty and then you're stuck with that reputation. It'll take years to get that back.

# Post-Show Blues

Competing is unquestionably difficult physically, but it's also a true test of one's determination, sacrifice, willpower, dedication, and patience. This sport can be more difficult on the mind than it is on the body. If someone isn't careful, things can quickly spiral downward.

It can be a mixed bag of emotions when someone decides to compete. One day it's great, the next it sucks, and people want to quit and then a couple hours later they're motivated again. It can most definitely be an emotional rollercoaster.

Eating the same things over and over again, plus daily cardio and weight training does get to be a lot. Then you have work, family, friends, and life added to this recipe and it can get quite stressful at times. There is one thing for certain though, the second you step on that stage after going though that tremendous mental and physical strain, it is all worth it.

Competitors have sacrificed and beaten themselves down physically and emotionally just to build themselves up again even stronger to walk onto that stage in the best shape of their entire lives (if done correctly). The feeling of euphoria in this moment is so powerful that it can be felt deep within your heart and soul. It's absolutely blissful. Even if you come in last, the accomplishment of going through the process is something to be extremely proud of.

These feelings are often short-lived. After the show is over, real life obviously has to begin again, and the adjustment can be very difficult for some. This is what is referred to as the *post-show blues*.

Life before a competition is so extremely scheduled and regimented that the sudden absence of this lifestyle can be quite a shock. With a ton of free time, less stress, and more money in the bank account, it can actually feel weird.

The main issue is trying to control the body's adjustment back to a normal diet. Obviously, prior to competing the diet is highly controlled and regulated. Dairy and gluten are usually completely cut out for months at a time, and the body has adjusted to this type of diet.

Adjusting can have its own array of challenges, and this is where serious eating disorders like anorexia, bulimia, and binge eating can unfortunately start to develop.

I remember my first two shows like they were yesterday. After they were over, I was actually embarrassed to walk down the chip aisle at the grocery store or even walk into some sort of fast food restaurant. I would cover myself up and look like I was going to rob the place to get a bag of chips from the convenience store. This wasn't a healthy mindset by any means. I've seen competitors refuse the leave their house or even want to go back to the gym because they feel "fat" or "ugly." Of course, this is never the case. Their minds have just adapted to seeing themselves shredded for months so looking anything other than shredded can be a total mind fuck. This needs to be recognized early so one can take back control and realize what is actually happening.

In my experience, women tend to suffer the most with post-show body dysmorphia. I'm not saying men don't suffer from it—they most certainly do—but women to tend to have a harder time with the adjustment back to having a typical body.

As competitors, we want to stay lean and look amazing, like we just hit the stage, but that's just not going to happen. We all know we need to feed our bodies and put them to work. That is how we achieved the look we had onstage in the first place. The second we steer away from that, we'll start losing what we have just accomplished. I feel some people forget what they learned about their bodies during prep and fall into the trap of "if I don't eat, I'll stay looking like I'm stage ready," or "if I just throw up after I eat, I won't lose this look."

This can become a downward spiral. You lose focus, gain a little weight, so you stop eating for a day or two because you think it'll get you back to what you looked like before. Doing that just slowed down your metabolism so when you eat again you start to gain more weight than expected, so you loop back into not eating again. It becomes a vicious cycle that can take you with relative ease if you don't realize what's happening.

Contest prep is hard. That's just the truth. When a show is over, many people want to look for an easier way to maintain that look. Unfortunately, there just isn't an easy way. It requires work and dedication to stay looking like an athlete. True athletes recognize this. If you gain a little extra weight, that's okay, just reset your diet and work the body a little more. Make the body work for you, not against you.

A lot of people tend to binge eat after a show, eating anything and everything they see. I've been guilty of this myself a few times. Since the body has adjusted to such a strict diet, binging can cause severe bloating, skyrocketing blood pressures, edema, and digestion issues. In some cases, people have gained more than thirty pounds overnight. I can see why the general public can think this is an unhealthy sport. In all honesty, if a competitor doesn't control their eating after a show, it can be unhealthy.

A lot of the weight gained from bingeing is water weight which the body is absorbing back into the system, but some is the body reacting to foods that it's not used to digesting anymore (mostly the dairy and gluten). When people get up the next morning they feel like crap, watered over, more bloated than a beached whale, and this is the start of the downhill post-show blues spiral.

This is when people feel that what they've worked for months on end has literally vanished in a blink of an eye. They just saw themselves onstage looking shredded, muscular and god or goddess like, but twelve hours later they look and feel like garbage, bloated beyond words. This can create a period of post-show depression that can become quite severe, leading to eating disorders such as binge eating, bulimia, or anorexia, as I stated before.

Bloating only lasts a couple days if you take back control of your diet, but unfortunately this doesn't happen all the time. Some people will go for weeks eating anything they want, but this only compounds post-show depression and weight gain.

This can be a learning opportunity for the future. This is a great time to learn about your body, for example, what not to do after the next show, what you can and cannot get away with in post-show eating, learning how and why your body has reacted in such a way, and what foods you are sensitive to.

After the show the body is fresh. It's like having a whole new body to experiment with and a whole new opportunity to live a healthier lifestyle. Even if you never compete again, use this newfound knowledge of yourself and integrate it into your normal daily life. If you do decide to compete again, you know what to improve on post-show to keep a better mental state to prevent the post-show blues.

A stage ready physique cannot be maintained. It just can't. When it's stage ready, the body is severely depleted and maintaining that depletion would be detrimental to your health. The body needs to get back to homeostasis. Getting back to training and keeping a balanced diet is the best way to help the body adjust back to normal in a healthy fashion.

Here is a little trick to help prevent major bloating and post-show blues. After the show, you can definitely have some junk food. Just keep it in moderation. Eat just one cheat meal, and don't drink gallons and gallons of water. Keep everything under control and in moderation. This is going to prevent that huge jump in weight the next day.

The day after you've had your cheat meal, get back onto your diet. Start dieting at about your eight-week-out diet plan. This will give your body just slightly more calories than it's used to, but not so many as to cause a lot of bloating. Keep up with cardio and training. At this point you're going to start feeling amazing. You'll be nice and full, but not bloated, and on the fast track to a heathy transition back to real life.

Slowly decrease your cardio and increase your calorie intake week by week. This is called "reverse dieting," the process of getting your body used to living a normal life again. This can be a slow process, but it helps prevent the dreaded post-show blues and post-show body dysmorphia.

If you are planning to continue to compete, there are other reverse dieting strategies to take in order to grow significant muscle mass, but that strategy is a bit more complicated and is something that needs to be planned and discussed with a good coach. For the athlete wishing to continue to compete, the first four weeks or so after the show is probably the most important growth period you can ever have. The body is at its peak metabolism rate, it's dropping fat like none other, and the body is incredibly anabolic. If you increase your calorie intake at this point, your body is going to soak them up like a sponge. This is why it's so important to stay eating clean after the show. You can't build solid muscle from poor nutrition. I won't go into more detail about this because this isn't a nutrition book, but if you want to continue to compete in this industry you need to know that this is the golden time period to get those huge gains.

Many people won't continue to compete after their first show. Maybe it was something to scratch off a bucket list, or maybe they can't take how hard the process actually is and they don't want to do it again. Who knows, but what is for certain is that competing is definitely not for everyone. If it isn't for you, that's perfectly fine. You tried something new, grew as a person, learned new skills, and had new experiences, and that is what life is all about.

Fitness, on the other hand, is for everyone. Competing is just one small part of this industry. Staying fit and healthy is something everyone needs to learn to do. This doesn't mean everyone needs to go to the gym, either. Hiking, swimming, running, playing hockey, football, or tennis is all part of fitness. Whatever gets the blood moving and muscles firing is perfect for long-term health. If you tried competing in bodybuilding and didn't like it, don't compete again, but don't let that steer you away from living a healthy lifestyle after the show or finding an activity that you truly enjoy.

# Chapter 4:
# The Ugly

**This chapter's special guest is Karen Harrison, ER nurse of over twenty years and my own mother.**

All sports have an ugly side, but it seems to be quite dramatic in bodybuilding. In football and hockey it's concussions, same thing with boxing and MMA. In baseball, it's torn rotator cuffs and knee ligaments; and in basketball it's mainly joint injuries. In bodybuilding, all of the above are issues. Add to all that steroid abuse and you've got a recipe for disaster. I've seen people drop weights on their faces, hands, and feet. I've seen people tear biceps, triceps, hamstrings, quads, pecs, and rotator cuffs right off the bones. I've seen people dislocate shoulders and knees. This doesn't include what happens to the inside of the body when steroid abuse is stacked on top of it. It can be a very dangerous sport if people aren't careful and taking the necessary precautions to protect themselves. Things like warming up, stretching, proper diet and rest, lifting with proper weight and form, being constantly willing to educate themselves on up-to-date scientific information and following proper supplementation protocols, etc., are all the athlete's responsibility.

This sport is changing constantly, and in order to survive it people need to be able to adapt and change with it. You need to adapt or be left behind. Education is a definite key to success in bodybuilding and fitness for both men and women.

# Steroid Abuse

What is the very first thing you think of when someone says "bodybuilding?" You likely do not think of health, longevity, community, or consistency. I can guarantee most of you went straight to steroid abuse. Unfortunately, this sport has an extremely bad reputation with steroid abuse, and with good reason. It has damaged the reputation of the industry immensely.

Notice how I said steroid *abuse*. That is exactly what it is. It's the abuse of these drugs that is the issue. Just like alcohol or many drugs, steroids can be used safely, but using them can get out of control very easily.

Steroid use is something you don't just dive into when you start getting into the sport. Steroid use takes serious thought and consideration. Many people start going to the gym and think they need to immediately start steroids. This is not true. There are many things to consider before starting a steroid cycle, and we'll go through some of them in this chapter.

What most people don't know is that when used properly, these drugs and the side effects are easily manageable, but it takes serious knowledge beforehand to know what you're dealing with and how to deal with them. Insufficient knowledge about steroids can lead to:

- the inability to be honest and open about the use of steroids because of society's stigmas around them;

- not regularly cycling off the substances to let your body heal and recover from their use;
- bumping up the dosages over and over again to try to increase your results because you have reacted well to small dosages.

Family and society that don't understand the sport often fear that steroids will cause death. You hear about people dying young that were using steroids. You're not always getting the whole story. There could be so many other components involved with most of these cases, but all you hear about is the steroids. You're only getting what the media is deciding to let you hear. They don't tell you about any pre-existing genetic conditions, other forms of drug use, circumstances leading up to the death, whether alcohol was involved or not, or if death by other means was a possibility or not. The second people find out someone who died was taking steroids, that was the automatic cause of death. I'm sorry, but that's just not the case.

I'm not saying that I think steroids haven't killed anyone. I do know that excessive and improper using can cause serious issues large enough to kill someone. Death can most definitely become a possibility if necessary precautions are not taken when using steroids. However, keep it in mind that steroid use isn't always the cause of death when you hear it from the media.

You have probably heard stories about young teens (not on steroids) dropping dead from cardiac arrest on the football field or on the ice while playing hockey. These sports take tremendous strain on the body as well, but hockey and football are viewed differently than bodybuilding. What I'm trying to get at here is that people need to open their minds to perspective and facts before assuming everything is blamed on steroids.

Fact: Cigarette smoking is the leading cause of preventable disease and death in the United States, accounting for more than 480,000 deaths every year, or about 1 in 5 deaths.[1]

Fact: An estimated 88,000 people (approximately 62,000 men and 26,000 women) die from alcohol-related causes annually, making alcohol the third leading *preventable* cause of death in the United States. *The first is tobacco, and the second is poor diet and physical inactivity.*[2]

Cigarette smoking and consumption of alcohol are legal. Why? I think we all know why. $$$$.

This is exceptionally interesting to me as it should be to you, too. Two of the three leading causes of death are legalized, while the second leading cause of death in the United States is what we're trying to prevent by going to the gym and working out. As a matter of fact, most people that I know who have started going to the gym or have started some sort of physical regimen have actually decreased their consumption of alcohol and/or cigarettes. Not only does physical activity decrease the chance of death from these three leading causes, it makes you healthier.

Steroids, like other drugs, have legitimate uses. Treatment for breast cancer, and help with osteoporosis and muscle wasting diseases are some ways steroids are used in the medical field. Sometimes steroids are even given to babies to help them grow if they are undersized. Steroids are clearly safe to use in these controlled environments if properly monitored.

Steroids is a multi-billion-dollar industry which means you'll be very surprised to know that a lot more people use them than you think. I'm not only talking about athletes, bodybuilders or people with specific medical conditions. I'm talking about

---

[1] U.S. Department of Health and Human Services

[2] Center for Disease Control and Prevention (CDC)

both men and women that are doctors, fire fighters, police officers, public servants, high school and college students, business owners, CEOs, laborers, etc.

One of my main goals is to open up the communication lines about steroid use so people can have the proper knowledge and support needed when using anabolic steroids properly.

Unfortunately, the fitness industry has developed to a point where people think that they have to start steroids the second they start going to the gym. Again, *this is not the case.* The absolute opposite is the truth. Being on steroids doesn't mean you're going to achieve great results. It takes way more work to properly be on steroids than it does to not be on them. There are many things to consider before starting steroids.

At the very basic level, anabolic steroids don't actually make you grow. They help you heal faster. When a person trains in weight lifting, muscle fibres tear at a microscopic level. That's why you feel sore after you lift weights or work out. This is a good thing. Now, recovery is necessary to heal from this. This healing process is actually how muscles increase in strength, volume, and size. The same process occurs when someone breaks a bone. When a broken bone heals, it becomes thicker than it was before, making it stronger.

Steroids help your muscles heal at an extremely accelerated rate. So, the faster you heal, the faster you can train again. The more training you do, the bigger you get. That is the very basic description of what steroids do, but people need to be aware of the downsides that come with it. Here is a list of some of those, not accounting for the actual side effects of the steroids. I'll get into those later.

- It is very expensive. To have a proper cycle (three to four months) for a beginner will cost about twelve- to eighteen hundred dollars. More advanced users and/or abusers can spend upwards of four- to eight thousand dollars per month. This isn't including a post-cycle therapy PCT protocol. I'll explain what this is later in the chapter.

- It takes frequent intramuscular injections. So, if you don't like needles, you're in trouble.
- If you don't keep to a tight schedule of when you're taking your dosages, you will not get the results you're looking for and could actually cause negative results instead.
- Your diet is extremely important when on steroids. Say goodbye to pizza and burgers. You need to eat lean and clean. I'll get into why when I talk about side effects.
- Your food intake is going to increase exponentially. Your metabolism is going to skyrocket (if you are using properly). Since people should be eating a clean diet, this is going to get very expensive.
- You'll need to invest in health supporting supplements. This means spending even more money.
- Since anabolic steroids are illegal without a prescription, you're going to have to be extremely careful about who and where you get it from. Just like other recreational drugs these days, people are trying to stretch their dollar and cut these drugs with really harmful substances.
- Someone is going to notice at some point that you're using steroids. Be ready to deal with that. Give them a copy of this book. It will help you open up and talk to your friends and family about these subjects.
- If you are on a steroid cycle and need to cross a border, it's always going to be a risk. Travelling anywhere is a risk while on steroids. Check your local laws on this matter. In most places, it is legal to be in possession of steroids for personal use. You can ask doctor for a prescription,

but you may have to just buy new steroids when you get to your destination.

Ask yourself if you are really prepared for this kind of commitment. Think it through. If you don't, you could be in for some very nasty and expensive surprises.

**Karen** - *"I was concerned about bodybuilding for a few reasons. It is notoriously linked with steroid use and abuse. I've seen firsthand how it messes with people's minds and bodies. I was scared that my son might get trapped or pressured into that part of it, and I didn't like that my son was going to be involved with the industry for this reason. I also was concerned that maybe my son was struggling with what his body looked like, as I have, for as long as I can remember. I didn't want that pressure and mental torture for him. I wanted him to be proud of how he looks and feel good about himself no matter what size shape or size he is."*

# Side Effects

Side effects can range in severity. It depends on a multitude of things, such as which substances are taken, and in what quantity, duration, and frequency. It also depends on the person taking them. Some people, like myself, can take these substances without serious side effects or issues, but I know many people whose experience is the complete opposite. We're all built differently, and we will all have different reactions to different substances. For example, one person can eat handfuls of peanuts while someone else might die just smelling them.

This is the main reason why it is extremely important to start with low dosages of only one or two steroids at a time. People need to know how their bodies are going to react before they get into more complex stacks and slightly higher dosages. Keep in mind that because your body may react well to a small dosage, it doesn't mean it's going to react well with higher ones. The body is very complex and even the smallest change can bring on big results or big side effects. *Be careful!* It should also go without saying that just because you react well to high dosages, it doesn't mean you should be taking such high quantities. That is drug abuse.

Here is a list of potential side effects of steroid use for both men and women:

- Insomnia.
- Night sweats.
- Acne (ranging from light acne to severe, whole-body acne).
- Oily skin and hair.
- Liver stress, which can turn into liver cirrhosis if not corrected. Liver cirrhosis is permanent liver damage.
- Kidney problems.
- Hypogonadism. This is when the sex organs provide little or no sex hormones (mainly estrogen and testosterone). For men, since the body has recognized it doesn't need to naturally produce testosterone anymore, the testicles shrink. In severe cases this can become a permanent condition.
- Clitoral enlargement. This is irreversible if not caught early. It can get to the point where a woman's clitoris looks like a small penis. In severe cases, it can get as large as a small thumb or pinky finger.
- Gynecomastia. Males start to develop breast tissue due to hormonal imbalance. It is commonly referred to as "gyno." In severe cases this can't be reversed and will require surgery.

- Erectile dysfunction.
- Infertility.
- Increased or decreased libido.
- Infection at injection points. This can be caused by not being sanitary while injecting, having bad steroids that haven't been manufactured properly, or an allergic reaction to one of the compounds in the drug itself. If not recognized early, this can be become life threatening.
- Baldness (men and women).
- Facial and body hair growth (men and women).
- Deepening of the voice (women).
- High blood pressure.
- Fluid retention.
- High cholesterol.
- Paranoia.
- Aggressive or manic behaviour. It is known as "roid rage."
- Ligament and tendon ruptures. The body is growing at an incredible rate, and the ligaments and tendons don't have time to catch up to the strength of the muscles. In some cases, this can cause them to become overloaded and tear right off the bone. This is actually fairly common. This requires surgery and will most likely end your competitive career.

Being in tune with your body is essential. It won't lie to you. You just have to be willing to listen to it.

**Karen** - *"When wrestling was a big thing in Calgary, many of the wrestlers were into juicing, even big name wrestlers such as the British Bulldog and the Harts. It was big business. I used to have to help drain the massive abscesses they got from injecting steroids, and I had to deal with their cockiness and moodiness. I was scared that this was the kind* *of shit my son would be exposed to and pressured into. I didn't want him destroying himself like they did. Most of them are dead now from complications from their careers, especially the steroid abuse. They ruined their hearts, minds, and bodies for what? This really freaked me out."*

Some of you may be thinking I'm just trying to scare you out of using anabolic steroids. This is not the case; I just want you to be completely aware of the risks involved. Just like every time you get into a vehicle you need to know that you might not be getting to your destination alive, or when you go swimming you could drown. These are real and potential scenarios, but they don't stop you from getting into your car or jumping off a diving board, do they? Why? Because you take necessary precautions to help eliminate those scenarios from ever happening. You look both ways at a stop sign before proceeding, and you make sure the water is deep enough before diving into it. Knowing the potential risks just helps you become fully aware of the situation and ready to combat anything that could happen. Failing to prepare is preparing to fail.

# Cycling Off Steroids

Even if you use steroids properly, eventually you will need to come off these substances to allow your body to recover before starting again. This constant on and off process is called "cycling." Cycling should also be used for stimulants, but that's for a later chapter. Cycling helps protect the body from long-term damage so you can maintain a long and healthy career in the bodybuilding and fitness industry.

A lot of people are unwilling to cycle the steroids; they are constantly on and are not letting their bodies recover.

Unfortunately, this can significantly compound the negative side effects, resulting in very serious medical conditions, which were listed in the previous section. Maximum recommenced cycles should range from twelve to sixteen weeks on and taking a minimum of eight weeks off. Off cycles can be worked around what is going on in life such as vacations, injuries, work schedules, etc.

For most people on steroids this can be very difficult. Steroids can make a person feel superhuman. They are stronger than ever, usually leaner than ever (If dieting properly, which they should be), and they have more energy and endurance. They heal faster, so there is less post workout pain, and usually users' sex drive increases through the roof. So, you can see why cycling off can be difficult for some people to wrap their heads around.

Cycling off is a necessary part of the process for a few reasons:

- It allows the body to detox from some of the harmful side effects and chemicals steroids can cause and have.
- The body is allowed to recognize that it has the ability to function properly without steroids. This is going to be very important when it comes time to come off steroids permanently. This can prevent permanent hormonal damage which would require injections for the rest of someone's life just to maintain proper hormone homeostasis.
- If an individual decides to start another steroid cycle, the body is going to be extremely responsive to lower dosages. This will help alleviate potential substance abuse, side effects, and significantly bring down the cost of using steroids.
- It keeps the body confused. The human body adapts extremely quickly to anything that it's put through.

This includes diet, training, and steroids. All these things need to be constantly adjusted to keep the body responding and growing to its full potential.

Post cycle therapy (PCT) is a drug protocol that takes place after a steroid cycle has concluded. The purpose is to kick-start the body back to normal physiological hormone levels as quickly and efficiently as possible. This helps eliminate muscle loss when coming off steroids, as well as keeps energy, bodily functions, and sex drive levels at an appropriate level. This can also assist one's mental state, by knowing that they have a substance that's helping their bodies reach natural homeostasis. Unfortunately, this doesn't happen overnight. This takes some time. If someone hasn't permanently damaged their body, it can take up to a year for the body to re-establish its pre-steroid hormone levels.

"Blasting and cruising" is when someone finishes a steroids cycle (blasting), but instead of performing PCT and letting the body fully come off the steroids, they lower the dosages significantly so the body doesn't have to go through the stress of going through a full off cycle (cruising).

This can have its advantages and disadvantages. The main reason someone would decide to perform and "blast and cruise" is if they are competing and have two shows that are too close together to fully cycle off properly.

For heavy users, the cruise can be a decrease before fully coming off the steroids, making it easier for the body to adjust its hormone levels before starting PCT. This type of cycling can be fairly costly if it's done on a regular basis.

Obviously, the body isn't going to be able to detox from these substances, which means the body will have to go through significantly more stress than it should. The body also won't respond as well to the next cycle, because it hasn't been confused enough. It still recognizes that steroids are in the system, and has adjusted to those substances. Also, side effects can become more of an issue and the risk of causing permanent hormonal damage does start to increase at this point.

It can be difficult to fully cycle off steroids. The difficulty is more psychological than anything, because that feeling of ultra-human strength and healing won't be as easy to attain. It can feel depressing if you don't fully understand the logic and science about what the body is going through and why cycling off is so important.

On the flip side, cruising can keep hormone levels a little more stable as opposed to coming off completely and proceeding with a PCT program. Mentally, this can be more comfortable for some people, but this type of cycling shouldn't be maintained or done on a regular basis. Cruising does tend to help with maintaining a little more muscle mass that was gained during the blast portion of the cycle, but this shouldn't be too much of an issue if your diet, training, and recovery are on point. This is another reason why mastering diet, training, and recovery before starting anabolic steroids is so important.

# Communication

If you are in a relationship, discuss the use of steroids before you start using them. Your partner must to be made aware of the potential health side effects as well as the financial, sexual, psychological and physiological impacts of steroid use.

The loss of sex drive can end a relationship very quickly. Just imagine this: You love your partner with all of your heart. You want to be with them, you want to have sex with them, and you want to please them how they want to be pleased but you can't perform. This has nothing to do with your attraction to your partner, but everything to do with how your body is reacting to the substances you have been taking. You don't want your loved one to feel like you don't want them and that you are not attracted to them anymore. If you are open with your partner, and they know that the loss of sex drive is a potential side effect, steps can be taken to prepare your partner and make sure they still feel loved and attractive. My wife and I discuss this side effect on a regular basis. We have to. There are certain points (especially in a contest prep) when our sex drives tank, and other times where our sex drives skyrocket. Some steroids can increase the sex drive dramatically, seemingly overnight. This can affect a relationship in a positive or negative way. Couples need to be prepared for these kinds of changes, and open communication is important.

It's no secret that finances are a major part of any relationship. Just imagine if you haven't told your partner you've start taking steroids. You're spending hundreds or even thousands of dollars a month behind their back. Not only that, but now you are eating more than usual. Your grocery bill is increasing significantly. Your partner asks why you can't afford to go out on a date, or why you can't afford gifts, or a night out. Maybe it's to the point where you are sacrificing your electricity bill because your income is now going toward something that your partner isn't aware of. Unfortunately, this has happened.

It takes hundreds to thousands of dollars a month to use steroids properly. Plus time off work for doctors' appointments, checkups, blood work, etc. Unfortunately, if you're trying to hide your use, you're probably not going to the doctor, or getting your checkups and blood work done. Which in turn means you're probably not using the substances properly, which increases the risk of side effects. Your partner will find out eventually. The truth will always come out and when it does, you'll be lucky to have a partner at all when it's over.

Little things that normally wouldn't bother you start becoming big issues, and you suddenly start getting upset over the smallest things. What's going to happen when an actual problem arises? Your partner doesn't know why you're acting irrational. They could think it's because they annoy you or you don't love them anymore, but in reality, you are having negative psychological side effects from the substances you're on. You will need to confess your steroid use to your partner and deal with the consequences, or you can continue and deal with the negative side effects and hope things don't get worse. I don't recommend the latter.

Whether you live with a partner, family or friends, or by yourself, it is important to let the closest people in your life know what you are thinking about doing. Being prepared will most certainly help with preserving your relationships with them if things happen to go sideways. It also helps keep you accountable. Once people are open about their usage, they aren't apprehensive to make doctors' or blood work appointments. Loved ones can help keep you on track with a proper diet and training, which will help eliminate a significant amount of any potential side effects. If you are on anabolic steroids and are not training or eating properly, you have no business being on them. Open communication is by far to best way to use steroids properly.

# When to Start Steroids

Weightlifting has been around for centuries and has been traced as far back as China's Zhou Dynasty in the tenth century BC. Bodybuilding in its popular form has been around since the

1890s. The use of anabolic steroids started around the 1956 Olympics, when bodybuilding was in its infancy. The point is, there hasn't been enough time to acquire the studies needed to determine what is the best age to start anabolic steroids if one decides to use them.

Using what we know about human anatomy might help us make our own conclusions on this subject. We know the male body matures from puberty between the ages of eighteen and twenty-two. For females it's between the ages of sixteen and twenty. We also know that the male body will continue to put on muscle mass well into the mid-twenties. This is when the male body has fully developed.

I truly believe that waiting to push the body to its maximum potential *after* it has fully developed is essential. Having natural, mature muscle development as a foundation for building more muscle, and having the muscle to fall back onto when steroid usage is completed is not only important for health reasons, but also for longevity and injury prevention. Also, this would significantly reduce the risks of screwing up one's natural growth and development.

If you want to build a sturdy building, you need a strong foundation. Don't weaken your body's foundation by starting anabolic steroids too early. Allow your body to naturally develop to its maximum potential first, and master proper dieting and training techniques before even thinking about starting steroids.

I'm not saying you can't lift weights while you are young; this is perfectly fine and acceptable. I'm stating that if your body is still going through its natural development, I don't think it's a good idea to start anabolic steroids if that is the direction you decide to proceed with in your fitness career.

What concerns me the most is someone starting on an anabolic cycle early in life, i.e., while they are still naturally growing. We just don't know enough yet about how it effects that body, and we won't know until the people who have done this start to get off the anabolics later in life. I see young athletes that are twenty or twenty-two years old that are massive professional bodybuilders already. Although I am completely in awe of their accomplishments, this means that they have been using anabolics for at least a few years by this point. I'm honestly worried for these people, and I sincerely hope that there won't be negative consequences for them starting steroids too early. I hope they live a happy, healthy, and long life, but I'm concerned that the opposite could very well be the case. The disruption of the natural growth of the body with supplemental hormones could cause serious issues in the long term. This would not only be devastating to the athletes themselves, but it will also contribute to the negative image of the sport.

# Shortcuts

Steroids should only be used to achieve a purpose or a goal. I get that people want to look good, be attractive and feel super-human, but don't we all. This can be done naturally if you're consistent, focused, and hard-working. What most people are using steroids for is to provide a shortcut and cut out the hard work it actually takes to achieve and maintain a high-quality looking physique. It might work in the short-term, but in the long-term, it will not.

Fitness requires consistency, dedication, hard work, and focus in both training and diet. When people try to cut these essentials by using steroids, they will always fail in the end. Either with negative side effects from improper usage (if they aren't working hard to use these substances properly, most of these people just increase their dosages to try to make up for the lack of work they are putting in, thus compounding the potential risks), or by not achieving the results they were hoping for.

If you or someone you know are using anabolic steroids, please make sure they are being used safely. I know there isn't an exact guide on which substances to take, the dosages, and cycle lengths. This makes it considerably more difficult to determine what works for a particular individual. Research is the key to success with these substances.

Steroids cannot be played with blindly. These are serious hormones that can significantly affect the human body, either positively or negatively, depending on your quality of research and how you use them. How your body reacts to steroid use could be different to how someone else's body reacts. So please don't be naive or dumb about it. Start low, start slow, and start smart. Use your brain.

Peer pressure can be overwhelming when you're in the fitness industry. Both men and women have to deal with it. You will hear comments like: "You should get on gear. You'll be huge." Or, "Just use this stuff, use this amount, you'll be fine." Or, "That's not enough. You need more." Let these comments flow into one ear and out the other. They may have found what works for them, but that doesn't mean it's going to work for you.

Diet shortcuts also don't exist. I can get myself into the low single-digit fat percentages when I need to for a show, so I know a thing or two about this subject. It surprises me how much I hear about people wanting to lose weight, but all they do is continue to cut foods out of their diets. particularly carbs and fats. I'm not going to go into great detail about nutrition, but this is the worst thing someone can do for long-term results.

Will cutting carbs and fats out of your diet help you lose weight? Yes, but only temporarily. What happens when you run out of carbs and fats to cut? Then what? Are you just supposed to not eat now? You might have lost twenty, thirty, or fifty pounds by doing this but where do you go from here? The answer is nowhere.

You may have lost all that weight, but you have now put your body into starvation mode, also known as being in a catabolic state. The body is starving for nutrients and its metabolism has completely slowed, so the second you reintroduce any kind of carbs or healthy fats into your diet you will gain more weight than you lost. The body does this for a very specific reason. It has been in starvation mode, and any food that is reintroduced is immediately going to be stored as fat as a protection mechanism just in case it goes back into starvation mode again.

The same concept is true when someone tells you that they just "can't seem to lose that last ten pounds." They have put themselves into starvation mode by shutting down their metabolism completely by not eating enough, and they will never lose that extra weight unless they literally stop eating.

In fact, the opposite is required to lose weight in the long term. People need to start eating *more*. Obviously, I'm not talking about candy, burgers, pizza, breads, and pastas. I'm talking about well-balanced meals with complex, low-glycemic carbs (brown rice, oatmeal, some potatoes, grains, etc.), healthy fats (avocado, olive oil, nuts and natural nut butters, etc.), and high quality proteins (fish, lean beef, chicken breast, eggs whites, tofu, etc.).

A well-balanced diet is crucial, but as with any type of weight loss, it needs to be coupled with exercise and calorie output or it will all be for nothing. You will still gain weight if you're not putting these excellent calories to use.

In very basic terms, your body is going to realize that it's not starving and that it's okay to burn body fat for energy. Since the body is now consistently getting the nutrients it needs and loves, it just says, "I don't need this fat! We're not starving anymore." This is when the magic starts to happen. The body at this point can now not only lose fat, but also gain muscle mass/quality. The body is now in a state of growth and repair while incinerating that unwanted fat. This is known as being in an anabolic state. You can actually lose body fat in a heathy way.

I've said it before—fitness is a marathon, not a sprint. It takes consistent hard work to get the body you desire. It's a lifestyle. It can be done, and people are doing it every day, but they are only achieving results by staying focused and working hard. I cannot emphasize this enough. By the time you finish reading this book, I hope you'll remember: "Hard work, consistency and dedication."

Unfortunately, most people want results *now* instead of working for it. Mainstream media and companies trying to make a quick buck know this, so they spread false information about pitiful nutrition and exercise. They are preying on people's lack of work ethic, dedication, and inconsistency to make themselves rich. Sadly, people are falling for it in record numbers.

Patience is a skill that is on the major decline and about to go extinct in mainstream society. Please do not lose this skill. Keep practicing it. If everything was easy, everyone would have six-pack abs, be rich, and own a yacht. The fact of the matter is, results take time. Don't lie to yourself. Life is about working hard for what you want and having the patience to get it.

If you want success with diet, exercise, and living a healthy lifestyle, patience and hard work are a must or failure will be kicking in your front door. Set yourself up for success. Believe in the process, and let it happen. Change yourself from the inside out. It took years to become how you are today, so it's naive to think that it all can change in a blink of an eye. It's going to take time. Let it. It'll surprise you how fast you can change yourself if you just let yourself go through the process and not worry about changing overnight.

# Steroids in Perspective

Let's put steroid use into the context of other substances we put into our bodies. We all laugh at those TV advertisements for certain prescription medications, because the long list of side effects, many of which are much worse than the actual conditions the drugs are meant to fix. In my opinion, those drugs can be more harmful than the proper use of anabolic steroids.

Alcohol is a substance that is commonplace and consumption of it is socially acceptable. It can be fine in moderation, but here is a list of side effects from prolonged alcohol consumption:

- Reduction in coordination
- Damage to different regions of the brain such as the cerebellum, limbic system, and cerebral cortex
- Weakening of the heart
- Increased LDL (bad cholesterol) and decreased HDL (good cholesterol)
- High blood pressure and irregular heartbeat
- Liver cirrhosis
- Type 2 diabetes
- Pancreatitis
- Nerve damage
- Ulcers
- Manic behaviour
- Memory lapses
- Increased fat
- Decreased testosterone levels
- Inefficient metabolism
- Prevention of healing and recovery

- Here is the list of potential side effects of smoking:
- Increased risk of stroke
- Increased risk of cancer (particularly of the lung, throat, nose, tongue, larynx, pharynx, stomach, and bladder)
- Tooth decay and staining
- High blood pressure
- Impotence
- Heart disease
- Osteoporosis
- Eye cataracts
- Macular degeneration of the eye
- Emphysema

It's not a secret that fast food isn't healthy yet millions of people a day, including children, are consuming it on a daily basis. For some, multiple times a day. Side effects of prolonged fast-food consumption include:

- Insulin resistance
- Bloating and puffiness
- High Cholesterol
- Shortness of breath
- Heart disease or stroke
- High blood pressure
- Weight gain
- Increased risk of depression
- Acne
- Tooth enamel erosion
- Increased risk of cancer

Some of these side effects are very similar to the side effects of prolonged steroid abuse. When you take a broader picture of health and fitness and give yourself some perspective, education, and knowledge, are steroids really the issue here? The real problem is the fact that most of the time steroids are being abused due to lack of guidance, support, and education.

I'm not promoting steroid use; I'm just trying to prove that steroids have a much worse reputation then they should. Of course, they can cause issues, but many other things that people consume in their everyday lives can also cause serious issues if not properly controlled.

It is possible to compete in the sport of bodybuilding without taking steroids. There are plenty of tested federations to compete in all over the world, and I believe tested federations will start to grow at a rapid pace here in the near future. However, just because someone is competing in a tested, or "natural" federation, doesn't mean they aren't taking steroids or cutting agents. Unfortunately, people are still using substances that they shouldn't be when they are competing in these natural federations. I know many people that have either used steroids in the past and competed in natural competitions or were taking banned substances while training for a natural competition. There are ways to cycle off substances without getting pinched, and ways to beat the lie detector test that some federations use on their athletes before they compete. It's going to take some time for these federations to get up to par with their testing procedures and eventually it will be a lot more honest.

If you're truly a natural athlete, you're going to have to work your ass off, but it's going to be worth it in the end. Trust me. I was clean for years and still beating people on gear, and that was a great feeling. You can absolutely enjoy a long and healthy career naturally. If you want to stay natural, then do it. Don't mess with steroids if you don't want to. They will change your life and you have to be ready and accepting of that fact.

# Chapter 5:
# The Process

Here is where I give a little sneak peek into the life of a competitive bodybuilder or fitness athlete. It will give you a general idea of what the whole process looks like from the start of off-season to the end of a contest prep. It'll help you realize how incredibly different and difficult this sport is compared to other modern professional sports. You'll see the highs and the lows that you will inevitably go through when preparing for a show, and see the dedication and the determination necessary to get through the process.

## Off-Season

Off-season is the time taken off between shows. When I say "time off," it actually doesn't mean *off*, it just means you're not in a cutting phase of your diet and training. This time is meant to grow, improve your weak points, and recover from the toll a contest prep can have on the body.

What you do with this time is very important. Most people use this time to relax, take vacations, drink, and eat crappy food before they hop back into another contest prep. This is exactly what *not* to do in the off-season. Don't get me wrong, take the vacation, enjoy some junk food now and then, and have a drink or two. That's fine to an extent, but doing it on a consistence basis will never get you closer to the physique that you are trying to achieve.

Goal setting is very important when making progress in your career. Your big accomplishments will be a result of all of your smaller victories compounded over time.

Your goals can be anything you need them to be. They might be benching 225 pounds for twenty reps, or squatting 315 pounds for four sets of twelve, or curling twenty pounds for fifteen. Maybe it's losing two pounds a week over the next four weeks. You can make them whatever you want, but when you make a goal, you need to be one hundred percent focused on that goal. Winning these small goals are incredibly important for your confidence. Bodybuilding is about training your mind just as much as your muscles, and this is a great way to do that. Constant confidence spiking will give you the faith that you're able to achieve even bigger goals.

Your focus, dedication, and consistency in the off-season are extremely important. This is where all your progress is made. This is where you work out your weak points, enhance your strong ones, and where mature, dense muscle is developed. What a lot of people don't know is that in order for muscle to mature it needs to be kept on the bone. Meaning that if you lose ten pounds of muscle and gain it again, it won't look hard and dense because that muscle is new again. If you keep that ten pounds of muscle on your body through the off-season, it will give that muscle time to mature, and mature muscle looks completely different than new muscle. It's more striated, separated, defined, and hard looking. This is the look you want when competing. You cannot be lazy when you're in your off-season. You still need to be consistent, focused, and dedicated if competing is something you wish to pursue in the long-term.

If you've done a proper off-season, you shouldn't need to be dropping forty or fifty pounds for contest prep. I have made this mistake a couple of times, and it is extremely hard on the body. When you have to lose that much weight in such a short amount of time, you will inevitably be losing some muscle mass with it. You've worked your ass off to build that muscle, so why lose it just because you couldn't control your diet and training in the off-season?

Also, when you start a contest prep within about twenty pounds of your stage weight, your energy levels through the contest prep are going to be incredibly higher. When you don't have to cut so hard, you can feed your body more. The more fuel your body takes in, the more energy you have. When you get to properly feed your body, you can actually gain muscle mass (to a point) while dieting down and leaning out.

You should be eating pretty much the same foods in off-season as you would during a contest prep, just in larger amounts. Of course, you can have your pizza, pasta, and burgers, but you must keep them in moderation. Your diet should be a minimum of eighty percent good, whole foods. This isn't without reason. You are building a sculpture to reveal to the world, and why would you want to build your sculpture out of shitty material?

You need to build your physique with quality nutrients, or you're setting yourself up for failure. Junk food tastes amazing; I love eating it too. I could eat it every day, but in this sport you don't eat for flavour, you eat for purpose and results. If you want results, be prepared to be eating the same things over and over again, so you'd better start getting used to it. Some tricks people use to make the food taste a bit better are adding hot sauce and seasonings. Some people like to use barbeque sauce, but the problem with barbeque sauce and anything similar to it is the amount of sugar it contains. You can quickly add

95

one to two hundred calories a day just by adding those sugary, carb-loaded sauces.

Remember, the types of food you eat are the materials you're using to build your physique. Contrary to popular belief, all calories are not the same. That means the IIFYM (If It Fits Your Macros) theory doesn't apply to the industry of bodybuilding. For example, three hundred calories of chicken and brown rice is totally different than three hundred calories of KD and hot dogs. The chicken and brown rice is full of protein, amino acids, minerals, and fibre, while the KD and hot dogs are filled with preservatives, sodium, and empty calories with no nutritional value. Also, the way the body responds to these foods will be vastly different. For example, the brown rice has a much lower glycemic index than KD (glycemic index indicates how much your blood sugar spikes after eating a certain food). Your blood sugar spikes significantly higher when you eat KD, meaning your pancreas is going to secrete more insulin, which means you're likely going to gain more fat, which means KD is not going to get you results.

Staying consistent on an off-season diet is going to make the transition to contest prep exponentially easier. There isn't a huge shock to the system, so the transition is smoother than a fresh jar of Skippy. Cravings are drastically reduced, and there is no real change of routine, thus reducing the stress of transition into contest prep life drastically.

Basically, it comes down to this. There really is no true "off-season" in bodybuilding. That's just one of the qualities that makes it the most difficult sport on this planet. When one show is over, you are immediately prepping for the next one. This is a 24/7, 365 days a year sport. If you want success in this industry, you had better start getting used to it. It's going to take its toll on your body. You're going to want to quit over and over again; you're going to ask yourself if it's really worth it. But at the end of the day, the iron runs through your veins, and you won't be able to live without it.

# Contest Prep

Now that you've worked your ass off in the off-season to get ready for your show, the time has come where things are about to get serious. Contest prep is a whole different beast when it comes to training, diet, and mentality. There is no room for error. These two to four months are going to be the hardest financial, psychological, and physical months you've ever experienced, so you had better buckle up and get ready for the ride.

This is when you start to deplete your body, tweaking your diet slightly to get you into a slight calorie deficit while at the same time giving your body the nutrients it needs to function. There is a really fine line here, and I've personally been on both sides of the fence. If you have too much of a deficit, you'll lose a ton of muscle mass and go into the show looking tiny, flat, tired, overworked, and be unmotivated to even step onto the stage. Having personally gone through this situation a couple of times, I would highly recommend postponing your competition and taking the extra time to slowly diet down. You'll feel healthier, you'll enjoy the process more, you'll keep most of your muscle mass, and you won't be as grumpy and moody during prep. There are so many positive aspects to delaying a competition to make sure your body is ready to show on stage compared to if it isn't. With all that effort, money, pain, sweat and sacrifice you put into it, why wouldn't you do everything you could to make sure you look the best onstage?

At the other end of the spectrum, if you don't have enough of a deficit, you won't come into the show conditioned enough. You'll still have fat and water weight on your body, basically making you look like a beached whale. Both of these scenarios can be extremely difficult to deal with mentally. You've worked all year for that show, and you failed at bringing in the best package you could. Again, I've also done this too.

It's not a failure if you learned something from it. Now you'll know what not to do, what your body is or is not capable of, and you can adjust for the next show. Don't give up because you lost. Even champions have lost shows. It's called paying your dues, and it's all part of the process. You cannot learn how to win until you've learned how to lose.

Your body is always changing and it isn't going to respond the exact same way with every prep. Having the ability to recognize these changes will give you an advantage against your competition. The only way to figure this out is to compete multiple times. Consider it as practice to figure out how your body operates. You'll learn which foods your body likes and which it doesn't, the amount and timing of your meals, how your body responds to different types of training and cardio, etc. Note these things in your first few preps so you're ready to nail the preps after that. Patience is absolutely key here. You need to constantly be open to learning new training and dieting concepts to see what works best for you. It takes some practice but you and/or your coach will figure it out if you really want it.

Your training will change during prep. You won't be lifting as heavy, because depletion takes a toll on the body, and you will inevitably lose a little bit of muscle. It just happens, even on steroids. Less muscle means the amount of weight that muscle can lift will decrease. Therefore, this is the time to start to define and condition your muscles. It's not about building tons of mass at this point, it's about shaping the muscles and conditioning them to "pop" when you flex them onstage. This usually requires higher rep ranges, stronger holds at each muscle contraction, and long, hard negative reps. You can't do this with heavy weights.

When you're in a state of depletion, aka a calorie deficit, your body isn't fueled enough to lift heavy weights on a regular basis. It's also really tough to lift heavy when your output is increased with cardiovascular training. When you start to deplete the body to become more defined, dry, and harder looking, your ligaments and tendons and more prone to injury. This is more of an issue for athletes on steroids, but it can become an issue for natural athletes as well.

Prep is the time when you really have to start nailing down your posing and determining what your strongest and weakest poses are. Bring your weakest poses up to par. Constantly practice your posing. You're going to be so depleted when you're onstage that the less thinking you need to do the better. Your poses should become muscle memory by the time show day arrives. The last thing you want is to forget how to pose when you're onstage. At every show, there is always one person that forgets, so make sure that it's not you.

The further you get into prep, the more you're going to notice that you'll start accidentally doing some weird things. Like putting your eggs in the pantry and your protein powder in the fridge. Maybe even adding oatmeal to a boiling pot of water instead of rice. These little mishaps are from what we call "prep brain." You start to forget simple things, become a little clumsier, and sometimes you can forget how to say words. Don't worry, it's normal. It's just what happens when you start to put your body in a depleted state and your brain is literally running on fumes. This affects some people more than others, but it'll go away the moment you get a re-feed (a calorie spike to keep your metabolism running at a high rate) or when your show is over and you get to start to eat like a normal-ish human being again.

Contest prep is mentally exhausting. Your mental capabilities are being put to the test. The further into prep you get, the more tired you become. The ability to push through your workouts, eat your meals, and even finding motivation to get out of bed will be difficult.

Working on prep is definitely difficult, and what you do for a living can make it even more of a challenge. For example, if you're a first responder and you're on contest prep, you still need to perform at one hundred percent at work, because people's lives are at stake. This can most definitely be stressful and extremely difficult. If you have to travel for work, having to plan ahead for your meals and training isn't going to be fun, let alone having to work on top of that. Unfortunately, your work performance is likely going to suffer a bit, so communicate this with your employer. Being open with them about what you're doing is the best way to keep things in your work life in good standing during prep.

At points your mind may start to fuck with you a bit, making you think that you're not going to be ready for the show. This happens almost every time I complete, even when I'm in phenomenal shape. In the back of my mind, however, I know I'm going to be ready. A lot of fitness athletes have similar feelings closer to show. I believe it stems from always wanting to be better, always wanting to be the perfect image of what we've imagined ourselves to be. It's just our competitive minds messing with our emotions, and being in a state of depletion makes us a tad more emotionally vulnerable. You have to push through these thoughts. You agreed to this, now keep that promise to yourself and push though. Then you will prove to yourself that you are capable of anything.

Bodybuilding and fitness is just as much about staying in tune with your body as it is about training and dieting. Listening to what your body is trying to tell you is a crucial skill that is often overlooked in the industry. It takes practice and consistency to really know how your body responds and to figure out what your body is trying to tell you. The more you learn and acknowledge what your body is trying to communicate to you, the better you can adapt your training and diet to get the best possible results. This includes knowing when to train certain body parts, when you need to take a rest day, when to time your meals, and what foods your body needs at a particular time.

The last week of prep is where things start to get exciting. You're so close to the show and you are looking phenomenal, but this week can also be the hardest. This week is all about depletion. I personally hate peak week, but I know people that love it. It's all super high reps training with almost no rest, so as to deplete as much glycogen out of your muscle tissue as you can. Then you get to start to re-feed your muscles with carbs again, to fill out and get that super tight look to your physique. Push through it. It's the last week. You're so damn close. When things start to get tough for me, I take one day at a time. If I can conquer one day, I know I can conquer the next, and the next day after that.

Stay as consistent as possible. If you miss a meal or have to miss a training session, let your coach know and get back on track immediately. Your coach needs to know so they can make necessary adjustments. If you keep screwing up, the chances of you placing well will start to decline, and that's on you. Personally, I'd rather not screw up anytime during the prep, that way I know I did everything I could to place well. There are no "what if" questions such as, "What if I just ate the meal?" or "What if I didn't miss that training session? Would I have placed better?" or "What if I didn't eat those extra cheat meals? Would I be leaner?" Eliminate those possibilities from the get-go by just getting the job done. No excuses. Making every day a win will lead to the big win when you walk on that stage, whether you win that show or not. You have proven to yourself that you can push though the hardest four months of your life.

Once you get to about twenty-four to twenty-eight hours before your contest day, you need to think about shaving and/ or other methods of hair removal. For me, shaving is the easiest, most efficient, and cost-effective way of hair removal. You need to shave so you your muscle definition can be seen, and so the spray tan you're going to get at your show has something to stick to. It needs to stick to skin and not hair. Here lies the annoying part, though. Once you get contest lean, shaving can become a real pain in the ass because you have all these new crevasses to shave into. For example, shaving in the armpits can be difficult. If you have deep-cut abs, those can be a pain in the neck to get into as well. Not only are these newfound crevasses a pain, but shaving where you can't see is a task of its own. Personally, I get my wife to help me. I get her to shave my back, some places I miss on my arms and legs, and my ass cheeks. Yes, she shaves my ass. Just the cheeks though, no crack action. I recommend asking someone that really loves you for help with this. It can be quite a bonding experience to say the least.

Exfoliating is extremely important, as well as not wearing any perfumes, colognes, lotions, or deodorants. If you get a spray tan with any of these things on your skin, your skin will turn green and you'll look like crap onstage. This could literally cost you your competition. Follow your tanning guidelines exactly. This cannot be emphasized enough. Don't ruin your show because you couldn't follow some very simple tanning guidelines. I've seen it way too often.

When you're competing, focus solely on yourself. Don't give your competition a second of your attention. Creeping your competition, especially on social media, can shatter your confidence and crush your self-esteem in a matter of seconds. People can get caught up with what their opponents are doing and how they are looking instead of focusing on themselves. This is a sport that requires you to be consistently beating yourself. You are your own competition, always. If you focus on someone else, you're going to pick yourself apart. "My biceps aren't as good as his," or "My glutes aren't coming in as much as hers are," etc. Everyone is different. Just because someone might look good halfway through their prep doesn't mean that they're going to look good on show day. The opposite is also true. Just because someone doesn't look good now doesn't mean that they're not going to look killer onstage. This puts unnecessary stress on yourself. Stress causes increased cortisol levels, and that means less fat loss, poor recovery, and less muscle gain. So really, you're just sabotaging yourself by creeping on your competition. Just be the best you can be.

Lastly, you must be all in. You can't have one foot in and one foot out of the door with this process; it's one hundred percent or nothing. If you're not all in, just stop while you're ahead and save yourself the money, the sacrifice, the pain, and the headaches. When you're into competitive fitness, you'll quickly learn if you have what it takes. Contest prep will hit you in the ass harder than a freight train if you're not ready and fully prepared.

# Contest Day

You did it. It's time to compete. All your hard work is about to come to fruition, and now it's the day before your competition. One thing to keep in mind is just because you are less than twenty-four hours away from your competition, it doesn't mean you can lose focus. Many first-time competitors make the mistake of taking their foot off the gas at this point in the prep. You're not done focusing until the show is over.

I've seen people start eating cupcakes, bags of chips, and chug litres of water before they walk onstage, and it completely destroyed all their hard work. People who looked like they would have placed first or second didn't even make the top five because of this simple mistake. *Do not lose focus.* It is extremely important to stick to your plan to a tee.

A little trick I have learned is when you're booking your hotel room, request a microwave in your room or bring your own. It's going to make your last meals of prep remarkably more enjoyable.

The day before the show is going to be nonstop busy. You'll have the athletes' meeting to attend where they go over contest rules and height and weight checks for all categories, as well as how the contest is going to be run the next day. You'll also have your spray tan and constant check-ins with your coach (if you have one, which you should). You're not going to get much downtime.

Your spray tan is going to be an interesting experience if you haven't had one before. Women usually get tanned naked, while men will usually wear a sock over their manhood. The sock tends to want to fall off, so sometimes you end up getting tanned naked as well. Guys, be prepared, because you'll be asked to move your junk to the left and right to get the spray tan inside your legs. The last thing you want is a dick-shaped shadow on your leg when you're onstage (if you're a body builder that has to wear a mankini).

Whether you're a man or a woman, you will most likely be tanned by a woman, so also be prepared for this. Yes, you're going to be standing naked, or close to it, with a stranger all up in your business. Keep in mind that they are tanning hundreds of athletes in a span of twenty-four hours, and they will be tanning them again the day of the show for touch-ups. This is a huge task, and they deserve your complete respect.

After your tan, it is extremely important to wear loose clothing. My best advice is to wear loose underwear and/or a loose robe. Loose sweatpants and a baggy T-shirt will do as well. Wearing tight clothes will ruin your tan.

Here are a couple of tips to keep your tan looking its best. Sleep wearing loose, long-sleeved clothing and wear socks on your hands. If you don't, and you sleep with your hand against your skin, you'll end up with a nice handprint on your body that you can't get rid of. This is obviously not a good thing. Also, bring black sheets and pillowcases with you to the hotel and replace the white hotel sheets with the black ones. This is to prevent your tan from staining the hotels sheets because if you do, they will charge you for them and they are expensive.

When you need to go to the bathroom, hover. Do not sit on the toilet seat. The last thing you want is a toilet seat ring around your ass when you're onstage. For women, bring a pee cup. I know this is a little weird, but it works. Hover over the toilet and pee in your pee cup. This will prevent you splashing on yourself and wrecking your tan. Just make sure you don't put the cup on the counter so people that visit the room don't think it's a drinking cup.

Most people get their hair and makeup done right after their spray tan. Mainly women get this done but guys, I highly suggest you get some makeup done too. It'll get your face to match the colour of your newly spray tanned body, and will also prevent your face from looking super shiny under the bright stage lights.

Okay, you're checked in, tanned, and you've attended the athletes' meeting. Now it's a waiting game. You'll be checking in with your coach every couple of hours to see how you're doing and looking. Constant adjustments are going to be made to keep you looking your best. You probably won't sleep this night. You'll lie in bed with your eyes closed, but sleeping doesn't really happen. You'll probably be getting up constantly, checking in, and you're excited that it's show day.

You get out of bed the morning of the show and wait until it's your time to get your second coat of spray tan, then you'll head backstage. You are still checking in with your coach, making sure everything is still going to plan while preparing for your time onstage. While you're backstage, just relax. Chat with people if you like. Some people chat, other just lie down with their legs up while listening to some tunes. It's the clam before the storm, so enjoy this temporary moment of relaxation and peace.

About fifteen minutes before showtime it will be announced that your class will start pumping up. This pump up is to get blood flow into your muscles to make them pop, just like you would when you're training at the gym. Don't overexert yourself here; just get some blood flow. You don't want to start sweating when you're pumping up, or you'll ruin your tan before you even hit the stage.

At this point, your competition will start taking off their shirts and sweaters and you'll start looking around at everyone else's physiques. You might start comparing yourself to others, and the head games begin. You need to stay in your lane and focus on you. The second you let your mind wander while looking at someone else's physique, you become vulnerable. It's easy to be taken advantage of at the show. Since confidence is a huge asset, stripping that from yourself or letting someone else take it from you can give your opposition a huge advantage. Remember, you worked your ass off for this. You put in the work, and you look phenomenal. Don't let negative thoughts take the podium away from you at the last second.

The stage manager of the show will call your class to line up backstage before you're called up to present yourself. This is the moment you've trained for, so enjoy it. This moment when you're standing in line backstage is a whole ball of mixed emotions. It's excitement, fear, glory, sadness, happiness, and relief all at the same time. It's the most unique feeling I've ever felt.

When your name is called, walk onto that stage like you own it. The judges love that confidence. You need to be confident; you look like a champ, so act like it. Head up, chest up, and show the hell out of that package you brought to the show. If this is your first show, this can take some practice. Remember that you're being judged from the second you step foot on that stage to the second you step off it. You have to keep your head up, and never let your poses and posture collapse. You must stay strong and smile for the entirety of your time onstage.

It'll be difficult. You're riding the fine line of depletion. If you're riding that line a little too hard, you might start shaking when you pose and you can lose focus. Controlled breathing and relaxation techniques are your best defense if this happens to you onstage. I've even seen people faint onstage. This isn't good, but it happens. Pushing the body to the extreme can have consequences.

I remember my first show. I was holding back tears because I just completed the hardest thing I've ever done in my life. It can be nerve-racking, but hold it together until you're offstage. You did it. You trained your ass off, and owned that stage. It doesn't matter if you placed or not, you should be proud of yourself. Whether it's your first show or your twentieth show, you have just proven to yourself that you are capable of so much more than ever before. And whether you compete again or not, use this experience of consistency, discipline, and dedication and apply it to your everyday life.

# Post-Show

The show is officially over and your contest prep has come to a conclusion, and this is when things can go extremely sideways for some competitors. A lot of competitors have booked photo shoots for after the show, but they still go to the closest burger joint and chow down on a few burgers and get half cut on a single pint of beer. They wake up the next morning bloated because edema (water weight under the skin) has set in, and they have pretty much ruined their photo shoot.

If you've worked for months to look like you did onstage, don't fuck it up because you can't keep junk food out of your mouth for a couple more days. I'm not saying you can't have a little cheat meal after the show, but keep it small and light. You don't want your body to rebound like a yo-yo. It can destroy people's mentality and self-confidence in a matter of seconds, and it happens all the time.

Realize that you have slowly depleted your body to a state where it looks absolutely stunning, and it's going to need time to bounce back to normal. This means slowly reintroducing foods back into the diet in a regulated basis. Also, just so you know, post-show is when your body is the most anabolic. It wants to grow like crazy. So, if you are looking to add in some serious lean muscle mass during your post-show anabolic phase, you've got to feed it with solid, nutrient-dense foods like I have explained in the previous chapters.

If you are serious about this sport, post-show nutrition is just as important as contest prep nutrition. It literally never ends. If you just want to do one show, then you don't have to worry so much about your post-show anabolic growth, but you do still have to reverse diet out of your show so you don't cause yourself physical and psychological stress, which can be serious if not monitored properly.

# Chapter 6:
# For Friends and Family

**This chapter's special guest is once again my mother, Karen Harrison.**

The potential damage of not supporting a friend or family member who is even somewhat serious about this sport will push them away faster than you can imagine. I know this not only from experience (obviously, my mother isn't one of those people), but also from witnessing it happen to others. I have personally been through this painful process, and I continue to deal with these kinds of situations, even with my growing success. It is honestly one of the hardest parts of being in the industry.

The love for this sport runs deep in the heart and soul of a person. With the amount of dedication and effort it takes, it has to. Almost every athlete I know in this sport would be willing to die inside that squat rack or on the bench press because of how happy it makes them feel. I am one of those people. So, when there is risk of someone or something taking that away, it can feel like I'm being torn from the inside out.

**Karen -** *"Seeing my son have a purpose and that he is doing something he loves is the most positive thing. The benefits that he's fit and healthy to go along with it is even better! I think he has learned a whole new career and can do other things along with it like coaching, personal training, etc. The fact that he found someone to love who is also involved in it and understands it is a great thing too! His happiness is the most important."*

It's honestly less painful to leave a family member or friend behind than continually listen to them try to talk you out of the sport you love. We can't be around that kind of negativity or attitude if we want to make it in this industry. I've unfortunately had to push close friends and family members out of my life for the sake of my happiness and career.

I believe most of the abrasiveness of family members and friends comes from the fear of their loved one not performing the sport safely. This is their loved one we're talking about. Of course, they don't want them to get hurt and destroy themselves. I don't want that for myself either, or for any of my own loved ones, whether they are in the sport of bodybuilding or not.

If you have a loved one who is starting to be involved with the sport of bodybuilding, my recommendation is to learn and grow with them. Help them research proper training techniques and different ways to shock the body. Help them understand proper nutrition and supplementation regimes that fit their body type. Help keep them accountable to the process. Not only will this help them exponentially, but it will also help you become educated on all different aspects of the sport, easing your mind when it comes to the topic of bodybuilding. Most people don't fully understand or recognize the sport in its entirety, and that is where a lot of the hesitation comes from. Start learning. You might realize that it isn't as bad as you think it is. It takes some time and education but, in the end, you will be more comfortable with the sport once you start to understand the fine details, dynamics, and science around it.

**Karen** - *"Time made it easier. I needed to learn a bit more from my son and realize what it really meant and that it is a sport, not just a vain thing guys do. Knowing he was doing it safely, like with trainers and in a team, made me feel better too. His safety and health is really important to me."*

Imagine that you love something with all of your heart (it could be baseball, knitting, writing comic books, painting, or whatever) and someone you love dearly is constantly trying to take that away from you because they don't believe in it. You probably wouldn't want them around either. It's exactly the same concept as with bodybuilding. Honestly, I believe it boils down to selfishness, though I don't believe it's intentional. Obviously, family and friends want what is best for their loved one. Who doesn't? But at the same time, who are you to determine what is best for them? Your loved one is the one that gets to make that decision.

I know this might feel like a slap to the face and you might be reading this saying to yourself, "Who do you think you are to know what's best for my friend/daughter/son/husband/wife?" Of course, I don't, but I do know that your loved one knows themselves better than you do.

Okay, let's turn this around. Let's say the pressure you created for your loved one made them quit something they love. You're happy that they listened and you're assuming that everything is normal and fine. You continue to live your life, proud and ecstatic that your loved one listened to you. However, whether it's in a month, two years or ten, resentment in your loved one will have built up and will come out and likely ruin your relationship anyway.

You really have two choices. One, support your loved one in the sport, let them thrive, and if they decide it's not for them, then it's their decision. There are no hard feelings and they can happily move on. Or two, you pressure them to quit. They will always live with thoughts of "What if." "What if I didn't quit? What if my friends and family just supported me instead? What if fitness was something that I was meant to do but now that opportunity is over?" I know from similar experiences that these thoughts are torture. They can shred a person's emotional state into pieces. Your loved ones might never admit it, but this is where the resentment comes from.

Personally, my happiness is the most important aspect of my life. As should it be yours and the happiness of your loved ones, too. If I really had to, I would have cut my entire family out of my life without hesitation if it meant keeping my happiness. I am so thankful that was never the case, but I have had to sacrifice a few relationships. Honestly, having most of my family on my side has made a massive difference in my drive and determination in my success in this sport. Like I said, I would have done it without them, but obviously having their support makes it easier and it's definitely the way I would prefer to have it.

> **Karen** - *"I initially thought it might be a phase, but seeing how focused, driven, and disciplined my son was made me proud of him, no matter what he achieved in it. I also wished I could be that disciplined with my own self! Kind of jealous! I'm just happy it makes him happy and it's what HE wants to do. I will always be proud of him no matter what he achieves in bodybuilding."*

Weightlifting and bodybuilding can be a legitimate way to earn a living and build a life, especially for someone who is fully supported and dedicated to the sport. And as has been discussed throughout this book, bodybuilding can be extremely difficult on the body, and just like in any sport, injuries happen. Don't let an injury of a loved one in the sport give you permission to try to convince them to stop. For some reason, society thinks that a bodybuilding injury is completely different from an injury in other sports. Sports in general have the potential for injuries. This includes hockey, baseball, football, soccer, tennis, golf, etc. You probably wouldn't tell your son or daughter to stop playing hockey after they got a puck in the face, or quit football if they broke an arm or a collar bone, so please do not try to make an injury into an excuse to pressure a loved one out of the sport of bodybuilding.

If in five years your loved one doesn't want to pursue a career in the sport anymore, great. Now all parties are aware of what it involves, and at least they lived the last five years fully supported, happy, and loved by everyone around them. They can then move on to other things knowing that the people closest to them will always love and support them no matter what, and bodybuilding was not the life for them and they can check it off their list. Even if they decide that bodybuilding isn't what they want to do, it has taught them dedication, extreme work ethic, and consistency. These three qualities alone will help them tremendously with anything else they want to pursue in their lives. In the end, it will make them a better worker, family member, and friend, and you will be thankful for it.

**Karen** - *"For the families, hold your judgment for a while. I had assumptions that were all wrong and I learned that it isn't all bad. See what's happening with it and go from there. Be patient; it takes time for your beginner to get a routine down."*

# Chapter 7:
# The Client/Coach Relationship

**This chapter's special guest is Ryan Richardson, the head coach and owner of Team Ignite Fitness. (Instagram: @teamignitefitness)**

I highly recommend finding yourself a good quality coach when you're ready to take things to the next level. It seems like today everyone is an online coach or an "expert" in the industry. I'm here to tell you that this is absolutely not true. (This coming from a guy who also coaches.)

If someone has only competed in one or two shows, they are not ready to be a coach. It takes many years of knowledge and experience just to even think about being a coach. Be extremely cautious when trying to find a coach, because they will literally have your health in their hands.

Remember when I was talking about how small this industry is and how fast word travels? Over time, you'll hear about who the good and bad coaches are. Take your time. You need to do your research before you hire someone. You do not want to hire an inexperienced coach without doing your own research, blindly follow them, and end up with permanent metabolic damage or in the hospital. All of which has happened and is more common than you might think. Here are some things to help guide you to finding a good quality coach.

First, not only is experience a huge component of how good a coach is, but communication is also of the upmost importance. You need a coach who will communicate with you and answer your questions in a timely manner with clarity and reasoning. Keep in mind that a coach has to be willing to work with you as well. There are a few things that need to be discussed and proven in order to validate that you are a worthy competitor to be taken on as a client. If a coach doesn't feel like you're a right fit for them, they will not take you on as a client. I have personally done this myself with clients.

Here are a couple things to look for and ask when you're searching for a truly qualified coach:

- Have they competed before? How many times?
- For how long have they competed?
- What were their placings?
- How long have they been in the industry?
- How many athletes do they coach?
- What is the success rate of their clients?
- Do they have nutrition and/or training degrees?
- Is coaching a side job for them or is it a career?
- What is their experience and knowledge on performance enhancing drugs?
- Are they pushing their own steroid brand? If they are, be careful. They may just be trying to get more money out of you. Just because they may be a good coach doesn't mean they have good steroids. On another note, they may have access to good steroids, so you're going to have to ask questions about this.

Once you think you've found a good coach, start digging a little deeper. Start contacting some of their current and past clients and ask them some questions. Social media is usually the easiest way to do this. Just send a few DMs, and most of them will get back to you. This is going to give you a complete picture of what the coach's skills and knowledge actually are. It's also going to determine if that coach is blowing smoke up your ass just to grab your hard-earned money. Here are some questions to ask these competitors:

- What is their confidential opinion of that coach?
- How was their health after competing?
- How long have they been with that particular coach?
- What did they like and dislike about that coach?
- If that coach is supplying PEDs, did they have any side effects?
- Have they suffered from metabolic damage?
- Is that coach more focused on nutrition and training rather than drugs, or more focused on drugs rather than nutrition and training? (Hint: If a coach is more focused on drugs to get results, they are *not* the coach you are looking for.)

**Ryan** - *"You see drug protocols. Even just the lack of basic knowledge around the drugs. You go, 'What the fuck are you doing to this person?' Do your research, everything will tell you that this is so wrong, but half these people just put their trust in their coach. They'll never know they're doing something wrong until something goes bad."*

What's one of the biggest mistakes competitors make when finding a coach?

**Ryan** - *"The look of the coach. Here's the thing, I think it's a mistake on behalf of the person that's doing it. I think it's a great sales tactic for the coach, because there's so many people that fall for it. For someone actually buying a program though, I'd want to see what that person has produced."*

Is there anything that you look for specifically when taking on a new competitor?

**Ryan** - *"Past history. I mean, I have to look at the current shape, conditioning, muscularity, what class they're entering, and all that type of stuff. Someone who comes to me might look great genetically but has never been on a diet or followed a plan in their life and doesn't own a gym membership. They just have maybe a physically active job that keeps them in relatively decent shape for the average person, and then they come in and tell us they want to be a competitor. I turn them away every time. Let's start with an eight-week off-season plan, pick a later date, and see if you can handle it. I'm going to put you in the gym five or six days a week and I'm going to have you eating. You're going to be consuming calories at seven points of the day generally, five meals and pre and post workout. Don't overcommit. If you can do it and it works out, great, we'll put you into a show, but if you can't, then no. I've had to turn away multiple people for that."*

There is a rhyme and reason for this. Like I said before, bodybuilding is a lifestyle. People need to be prepared for how competing is going to change their entire schedule. Like Ryan was saying, start with an off-season plan first. Get your feet wet and see if you can handle it. You have to crawl before you can walk, let alone run. Contest prep is a whole other level of commitment. This will benefit both you and your coach. With a small off-season plan, you can see if this sport is something that you can handle before spending your hard-earned money on a contest prep. You and the coach will have the opportunity to work together to see if both of you work well as a team. The coach will get a good idea of how you are as a client, and you'll get an idea of how your coach is as a coach. Like Ryan said, do not overcommit when doing this for the first time.

**Ryan** - *"Start preparing to live a very, very structured life. Time management, scheduling. Learn the ability to stay very regimented, because the first thing when someone falls off track, they're not achieving results or things like that. For one, their time management sucks. They can't stay focused and can't stay on a consistent schedule. They're having a hard time trying to fit everything in and they just end up just saying 'Fuck it, I'm done.' We can get used to the food, we can get used to the training, we can get used to going to the gym, things like that, but when are you going to go to the gym? When are you going to meal prep? What times are you going to eat? Strategize a daily routine for yourself. I'd say that was the biggest thing for anyone just starting is realizing that their life has to take a lot more structure. I get people coming to me all the time saying, 'I don't have time to do this, I don't have time to do that.' Well yes you do, you're just not prioritizing them. There's always a solution for everything. Once you figure out a routine, stress reduces. You know what you're doing at any given time, you know when you're going to the gym, you know when you're meal prepping, you know when you're going grocery shopping, so if your buddy calls you or your mom calls you and wants to go to lunch with you, you know exactly when you can go. You don't lose your life. I think people get so overwhelmed with it* *and all of a sudden, they just collapse and feel like there's no time for anything else. You want to get into a contest prep, be prepared to make that your number one priority. So, you want to go to lunch with your mom, well, 'No I can't Mom, see you after the comp. Sorry Mom, come over and watch me eat chicken and rice.' That's the difference of how much someone wants to put into this."*

Let's say you've found yourself a great coach. They communicate with you, things are working out, and you're staying healthy. You did a great job with getting a coach, but are you a good client? This is a two-way relationship. Remember, your coach is a coach. You need to be completely honest and open with them about what you are doing. You can't hide stuff from your coach. This is the number one rule of being a good client. You need to communicate, too. Did you do more cardio than you were supposed to do? Did you have an extra cheat meal during the week? Did you miss a training or cardio session? Did you miss some meals? Are you getting constipated? This list of questions goes on and on, and your coach needs to know everything. That way they can adjust your plan accordingly to get you the results you want. You also have to be accountable and honest with yourself. I personally have a coach to keep me accountable to someone other than myself. That's just my style, and I work better that way. For whatever reason you get a coach, use them properly.

Coaches don't like to be pestered with texts and emails every five minutes. If you have a question or two, ask them, but there is a fine line between asking a question or two and being needy. Your coach is not your babysitter. Try doing some research first before asking a question. That way you can learn something for yourself and if you still have a question or want to confirm your research, then you can ask.

If you are not following your plan, a coach can fire you as a client. Whether you're paying them or not, you are a representation of their coaching abilities. Coaches want people to see the quality of their athletes. If you are risking that because you're not following your plan, then unfortunately that's on you. If you're consistently not following the plan, you're not only making yourself look bad, you're making your coach look bad too. Eventually they will fire you for that, and you won't be getting your money back.

However, it works both ways. If you're following the plan to a tee and you're not getting results, you can also fire your coach. Having a coach is a relationship and you need to work together. Sometimes things don't work out, or a coach and client don't jive on the same level. It happens. Just move on and find another coach that you think will be a better fit for you.

It's also okay to switch coaches if you want to. Even if everything is working okay with your current coach, sometimes it's beneficial to try other coaches to see how their training and dieting styles work for you. You might find something new about yourself with a different coach. Every coach has a different way of doing things, so it's possible you might get better results with one coach over another. This isn't personal at all, sometimes it's nice to try something new. If it doesn't work out, then go back to your old coach, as long as you didn't burn that bridge when you left.

As we discussed earlier, this industry can be extremely expensive, and these costs include coaching. Prices range from coach to coach, and they sometimes offer different services. For example, some coaches include posing practice as part of their contest prep packages and some don't. When you are looking for a coach, be wary of coaches who ask how much money you are willing to spend on their services. This is an indication that they're basing their prices on how desperate someone is. Unfortunately, this happens and, in my opinion, it is completely unacceptable. Athletes should be paying the same price for the same service no matter what their financial situations are. Just be careful.

> **Ryan** - *"Too many people give a shit about the bank account rather than the actual outcome of the client. They're focused too much on just getting that sale. I focus more on getting results with that person. That sale is now solidified and five of their friends are solidified. Put the focus elsewhere, and let the money come in later."*

Although bodybuilding isn't a team sport, it does require a team in the background for success. For example, training partners, coaches, doctors, HRT (hormone replacement therapy) specialists, good quality steroid dealers, and supportive family, friends, and partners are all part of your team. Having a high-quality team behind you is critical for your success in the sport of bodybuilding.

# References

Center for Disease Control and Prevention (CDC). *Alcohol and Public Health: Alcohol-Related Disease Impact (ARDI). Average for United States 2006–2010 Alcohol-Attributable Deaths Due to Excessive Alcohol Use.* Accessed January 18, 2017. https://nccd.cdc.gov/DPH_ARDI/ Default/Report.aspx?T=AAM&P=f6d7eda7-036e-4553-9968-9b17ffad620e&R=d7a9b303-48e9-4440-bf47-070a4827e1fd&M=8E1C5233-5640-4EE8-9247-1ECA7DA325B9&F=&D=..

https://www.alcoholrehabguide.org/alcohol/effects/

https://www.livestrong.com/ article/275029-the-history-of-weightlifting/

Mokdad, A.H., Marks, J.S., Stroup, D.F., and Gerberding, J.L. Actual causes of death in the United States 2000. [Published erratum in: JAMA 293(3):293–294, 298] *JAMA: Journal of the American Medical Association* 291(10):1238–1245, 2004. PMID: 15010446.

U.S. Department of Health and Human Services. *The Health Consequences of Smoking—50 Years of Progress: A Report of the Surgeon General.* Atlanta: U.S. Department of Health and Human Services, Centers for Disease Control and Prevention,

National Center for Chronic Disease Prevention and Health Promotion, Office on Smoking and Health, 2014. Accessed February 22, 2018.

CPSIA information can be obtained
at www.ICGtesting.com
Printed in the USA
BVHW061937140821
614237BV00003B/7